Sybil's Choice

Iris Sechriest

iUniverse, Inc.
New York   Bloomington

iUniverse books may be ordered through booksellers or by contacting:

iUniverse
1663 Liberty Drive
Bloomington, IN 47403
www.iuniverse.com
1-800-Authors (1-800-288-4677)

ISBN: 978-1-4401-6858-1 (sc)
ISBN: 978-1-4401-6857-4 (ebook)

Printed in the United States of America

iUniverse rev. date: 10/02/2009

Contents

What To Do (Or Not)
Sybil's fate is established

Oh, dear God, I still have painful regrets. Why did I? Should I not have? I? What else could I have done to make her last days better? There are so many simple things that, had I thought more wisely, I could have done differently during Sybil's horrific battle with an unrelenting malignancy. There are words I might have said, actions I might have taken or not taken, and deeds I might not have left undone before time robbed me of the privilege. I have no remorse, nor does anyone who loved her about agreeing with her major decision about her choice of treatment.

Even as tenacious tumors were spreading rapidly throughout her body, we truly believed that the tumors were shrinking. Our whole focus was on the cancer from the moment of that horrific detection.

I yearn to remake that period of our family history. And I so desperately want the ending to be different this time. My heart still pleads that it not be a true story but instead simply a tragic nightmare that eventually ends, and when it is over, I will be awakened again when Sybil opens my front door and spiritedly calls out to me, "Mom!" Then, with that frightening dream behind us, we will sit happily on my deck, chatting about our last "girls' night out" and planning the next one.

1

Fate, however, dealt a crushing blow to my child and our entire family. I know that it is not a dream, but cold reality. For me, it has been too unbearable to absorb all at once. It is a reality that will seep drip by drip into my very soul every day for the rest of my life.

The first hint of impending doom came with a casual announcement that Sybil made after she and her husband Bill had enjoyed a pleasant trout dinner in my small house. We were relaxing in the sitting room, watching the firelight dancing from small fireplace. Sybil sat across from me in a blue leather wingback recliner. She averted her eyes as she leaned forward to flick ashes from her cigarette into an ashtray on the side table. "I have an appointment for an MRI Friday morning," she said. Her tone was matter of fact, but the statement startled me.

"Wh—, what is going on?" I asked.

"Numb," she replied without wavering, as she passed her hand across the front of her lower body. I stared at her wordlessly while she sipped from her wine glass without offering further explanation.

I recalled the numbness in my arm and hand fifteen years earlier, symptoms of two deteriorating disks in my neck. After giving up on several months of chiropractic treatment, I had opted for surgery, which instantly eliminated the pain. With that memory in mind, I delicately suggested, "Maybe you have a pinched nerve."

She shrugged her shoulders. "I don't know. Guess I'll know after Friday."

"What time is your MRI?"

"Nine o'clock. Bill is going with me." He was silent during our exchange.

"Call me as soon as you know anything. I will be at Billy Joe's [Davis] office until 2:00 PM.

In retrospect, I wish I had said immediately, "I'll go with you," and that I had needed to stay with her throughout the testing and diagnosis. Of course, Bill was with her during the MRI, but as her mother, I should have been with her as well, and also through the follow-up with Dr. Godfrey. Thus began a series of missteps that often haunt me.

I am trying to forgive myself.

The call came through at noon on Friday. I had thought the MRI would probably reveal a simple explanation for her symptoms. Sybil was a lively, strong, healthy young woman. It was inconceivable that anything serious could be wrong with her.

"Mother, are you sitting down?" The tone in her voice was very serious, sobering me instantly. My heart sank.

"What did you find out?" Even as I asked, I knew I really did not want to hear anything dreadful.

"Bill went with me for the MRI, and afterward he went back to work. He'd just left the house when Dr. Godfrey called me from his office. Dr. Godfrey told me that there is a lesion on my brain." Sadly, I realized that she had been alone when she heard the ominous report. "And he has already made a Monday appointment with Dr. Steven Corso at the oncology clinic in Spartanburg."

I felt a hot wave of shock flash through my entire body, followed by a heavy sense of dread. Immediately my mind flashed to "cancer." That frightful realization eclipsed everything else. I did not trust myself to speak aloud.

After a pause charged with anxiety, I was jolted back into awareness when Sybil continued calmly. "Would you ask Billy Joe if our medical insurance covers this doctor?"

What could I say? A mother should have some words of wisdom to offer at a time like this. It is not simply a "kiss and make it better" kind of problem.

"It's the Palmetto Hematology Oncology clinic at Spartanburg Regional hospital" she added. Dr. Godfrey chose the Spartanburg hospital because of the urgency he recognized in Sybil's condition. The South Carolina facility would be the nearest facility available to care for her immediately.

Relieved to have something that would take me away from the phone for a few minutes, I responded, "Hold on, honey, I'll ask BJ." I pushed the hold button on the phone and took a deep breath in order to gain a bit of composure before walking into Billy Joe's office. As I passed the records rack on the wall, I pulled Sybil's insurance folder.

Billy Joe has been a friend of the family for over twenty-five years. He was one of Sybil's high school teachers, a big loveable man with a wonderful sense of humor. He sensed that something was amiss when I appeared before him, file in hand. He looked at me questioningly.

"Sybil has a problem," I said. I handed him the record as I recounted her information. BJ, with evident concern, assured me that her insurance would cover the cost of her care in Spartanburg. He and I made note of the address and directions.

The task of investigating her insurance coverage eased some of the emotional turmoil for the moment, and I returned to my desk and picked up the phone to reassure Sybil about her coverage. She acknowledged the information and quickly dismissed the topic.

"Don't forget about dinner tomorrow evening. Bill is going to make your recipe for trout. You can supervise him."

"Okay," I said lamely. My mind was still reeling from her shocking report.

"I'm going to tell Bill that I just want to be with family this weekend. We'll tell Randy to come without a date."

"I understand," I replied.

Family also meant Jayne, Sybil's college roommate. The girls were like sisters and talked every day on their mobile phones. So, naturally, Jayne would come from Rock Hill, South Carolina, for the weekend. Sybil especially needed her during this dreadful period. Best friends offer a magical perspective so different from what mothers can provide.

During dinner the next evening, we did not discuss Sybil's crisis as a group. But Randy and Jayne found a private moment to talk about Sybil's situation.

Jayne expressed her fear. "I just can't bear the thought of the dreaded *c* word."

"There's another *c* word to think about, Jayne," Randy told her. "The word is *cure*, and there is a *cure* for cancer," he said confidently.

Randy and his best friend Pat McEwen had done a tremendous amount of research on alternative medicine. When Pat's brother, Jim, was diagnosed with prostate cancer, Jim's oncologist told him that only radical surgery could save his life. He refused the surgery, and he and his family found an alternative treatment. They chose the Albarin treatment, which they discovered was undergoing a clinical trial in St. Petersburg and in Tampa, Florida. It was part of a three-year, federally funded clinical study. Albarin is a serum extracted from aloe vera. Jim began treatment immediately and soon saw positive results. The therapy successfully cured his cancer, and he continued to return periodically for maintenance injections. Meanwhile, Pat, who did not have symptoms of prostate cancer, chose to do periodic intravenous injections as a preventive measure. Pat is an airline pilot. Given his brother's diagnosis and the fact that airline pilots tend to be plagued with prostate cancer, he was wise to taking precautionary action. Randy was exploring the possibility of imitating his friend by joining the clinical trial for preventative therapy.

Randy's confidence and enthusiasm gave Jayne some reassurance, but she did not have the same blind faith in the aloe product that he seemed to have.

Later that evening, Bill and Sybil listened attentively to Randy's description of Jim's experience. In the days that followed, they also talked with Pat, who recommended other patients as referrals. When they spoke with the other patients, they were impressed. The information gave them another positive option besides chemotherapy to consider. That hope made Sybil's plight seem a bit less ominous.

Randy and I did our own research on my computer during the weekend, looking for information about Albarin. According to John Hammell, president of International Advocates for Health Freedom,

Research by the immunologist Ian Tizard, PhD and virologist Maurice Kemp PhD from Texas A&M led to the discovery that Aloe mucilaginous polysaccharide is taken into a special leukocyte, the macrophage, and this cell is stimulated to release messenger molecules, called cytokines (interferons, interleukines, prostaglandins, tumor necrosis factor and stem-cell growth factors).

Tumors release a chemical that attracts blood circulation so that malignant cells have a supply of nutrition and can keep multiplying. Tumor necrosis factor shuts off the blood supply to the tumor and it therefore dies. All of the immune modulating effects from Aloe contribute greatly to the prevention and healing of malignant cells. (http://www.iahf.com/usa/20011106.html)

The aloe vera cancer treatment involves an extract called Albarin serum, developed by Ivan Danhof MD, PhD. The serum is injected into the bloodstream to remove toxins from disease-fighting white blood cells. The treatment also raises the body's temperature, making it harder for cancer cells to grow.

Although we were gravely concerned, we were excited to find that there was a promising cure as an alternative. Randy went back to Blowing Rock where he would await the oncologist's diagnosis.

As I drove across town to my daughter's house on Monday morning, I was filled with dread. She and Bill were waiting for me to follow them to Spartanburg. The thirty-minute drive seemed to take forever. Then the sign, "Palmetto Hematology Oncology," loomed into view as I swung through an entrance behind Sybil's Buick.

Surprisingly, Jayne, habitually a latecomer, was there to meet us in the hospital lobby. "You're on time, Jayne," I remarked.

Her reply was an unnatural chuckle, "Yeah."

We waited in the middle of the room while Bill walked to the front desk to tell them that Sybil had arrived. We were told to wait in a nondescript room with bland walls and dark seating. The wait was much longer than the "shortly" we were told. Our intense dread made it seem much longer than it actually was. Because the MRI had revealed tumors, we all knew that we faced very bad news about Sybil. I tried unsuccessfully to drive the fear from my mind. *Don't think*, I scolded myself. My terrified thoughts were winning the inner struggle. My heart was sinking. Feeling sicker by the minute, I lamely attempted to make small talk, but that fell flat. None of us wanted meaningless chatter; nor did we dare mention our dread. We let the uneasy silence possess us until a grim-faced nurse beckoned us to follow her.

Dr. Corso, short, dark-haired, and rather handsome man, strode confidently to meet us in a hallway. His youthful appearance surprised me. We followed him through the corridor to where an X-ray was clipped to a display panel. He looked much too young to be an expert on a disease as complicated as cancer. Nonetheless, he spoke with credible confidence. Using a thin wand, he showed us an easily visible elongated tumor on the left side of Sybil's brain, and then moved the wand across to a smaller, barely visible spot on the other side. The picture clearly exposed Sybil's stricken brain structure.

"Come in and have a seat," he told us. He led us through a door on our right into his office. I took a seat in a wing chair beside a small lamp table. I noticed a framed photo of the physician and his family, a happy looking group, but I was already beginning to feel uncomfortable with the doctor. Jayne, Sybil, and Bill took individual seats to my left. Dr. Corso sat in a huge executive chair and spun sharply around to face us. His demeanor conveyed impending doom. My heart sank. The four of us stared directly at the doctor, as if to stop the words we knew would now come.

It was worse than I could have imagined. Speaking directly to Sybil with crisp authority, the doctor declared, "It is probable that you have brain metastases that arose from cancer cells outside the brain, more than likely in your lungs. We are going to admit you to the hospital for the night. I will schedule a CAT scan of your lungs early tomorrow morning."

Sybil stared at the doctor, gravely silent. I felt a chill run through my spine when he said lungs, horrified at the thought of spreading malignancy. Surely, she must have felt a similar hot streak of fright. Still, she said nothing. Neither did Bill.

Dr. Corso told her that other doctors would be involved: a brain surgeon, should the tumors we saw be operable, a radiation oncologist, and a pulmonary specialist, in case of possible lung malignancy.

He ignored her fearful silence and casually commented, "You probably want to go to lunch before you go to admissions."

Jayne shuffled her notes and turned to the doctor. "Can Sybil have a glass of wine with lunch?"

"Of course," he said as he rose from his chair, "she can have anything she likes." He was already turning away from us to attend to papers on his desk, dismissing us without another word.

It did not matter. He had said more than enough already. I rose unsteadily to my feet. We filed somberly through his office door toward the exit, craving a breath of fresh air to splinter the dark energy that emanated from Dr. Corso and his report. Indeed, once outside the dreary hospital walls, a crisp sunny day rewarded us with lighter spirits.

"Shall we go to Basil's for lunch?" I asked tentatively. "It's only a few blocks, just through the stoplight where we turned to come here."

"Yes!" Sybil exclaimed with enthusiasm.

Basil's Grill was a long-time favorite. Sybil and I discovered the delightful restaurant at their original location and later followed them a couple blocks down the street to their new location, which is larger and less intimate, but still a treat.

I was glad that we could share lunch at a place that I knew Sybil enjoyed. It was at least one bright event in the day's dramatic devastation. Because it was past Basil's normal lunchtime, there were patrons at only two tables; this gave us both privacy and fast service. We ordered wine and casually discussed the menu for a while, and then the conversation turned to easy topics.

"I've come prepared to spend the night," Jayne told us.

"Pajama party," I replied weakly. The only luggage I brought along with me was anxiety. "I'm glad you are going to stay."

What was there to say about the doctor's overwhelming information? The fact that we were mindful of Randy's information on an alternative treatment center preserved our mental state. Each of us had that unspoken anticipation.

As we were leaving our table at the back of the restaurant, Sybil swayed unsteadily and had to hold tightly to the back of Bill's belt for balance. The partial paralysis of her right leg was painfully apparent as Jayne and I followed the couple in a zigzag pattern through the tables.

Suddenly Sybil turned to two blue-haired women seated at a table against the wall. "It's rude to stare!" she said sharply.

Her instant anger and harsh retort shocked me. "What happened?" I asked, slightly embarrassed by her unexpected outburst. She had always been exceptionally friendly with everyone.

"Those two women were staring at me," she answered angrily when we had shut the dark heavy door behind us. I only saw them fleetingly, but I was sorely tempted to go back inside to denounce their attitude. I realized the incident was only one of many indignities my daughter might suffer in the future. Her hobbling gait was definitely that of a handicapped person (or, more politically correct, a "physically challenged" person). Such afflictions are a curiosity when the challenged person happens to be young.

Jayne and I waited in the main lobby of the hospital while Sybil and Bill worked through the annoying admissions process. When they returned, Bill led us to an elevator. I felt like I was sleepwalking when he pressed a button to take us to the cancer patient floor. Bill and Jayne were talking on the way up, but I think Sybil and I were in the same sort of mental stupor.

The elevator door opened into a luxurious space that easily could have been the atrium of an exclusive resort. Long planters filled with exotic greenery sat strategically along a protective rail in the center of the space, which overlooked the floor below. It was like walking into a quiet garden, at least until we saw a nurse's station beyond us.

Sybil's room was like a hotel room. Jayne deposited her overnight luggage in a closet beside a built-in shelf unit on one side of the room; the closet faced a large bathroom with a chair and handheld shower. We discovered a comfortable looking Murphy bed that could be pulled down alongside the patient's bed.

"Nice room," Sybil said, agreeably. She seemed to be facing her burden with stoic resolve. Nevertheless, I knew she was frightened beyond words.

I thought that surgery would remove the tumors. Surely the cancer could not have taken control so quickly. It must be in the early curable stages. *Oh, God, it has to be curable. It just has to be.*

A young nurse came in to check Sybil's vitals. Jayne and I watched her make cheerful small talk while she took Sybil's temperature; then she silently took Sybil's blood pressure. Bill in the meantime had been making calls to concerned family and friends who wanted updated information.

It hurt me to leave Sybil in the medical center that evening, with the uncertainty facing us. But Jayne was probably better company that night than I could possibly have been. It was becoming increasingly difficult for me to keep a positive look on my face. Her best friend, I thought, would a better companion than an overly anxious mother.

Once away from the hospital environment, I vowed to search for hope instead of desperation. The only thing I could think to do was to go back to the computer and search for more information on the aloe vera treatment as an alternative to surgery. Sharing that information with Sybil might give us both encouragement. This would become my salvation throughout the entire ordeal we faced: *a search for a cure, a search for hope.*

Morning found me impatient to get back to the Spartanburg hospital with the folder containing printed pages from my overnight research. I felt I had begun to understand the Albarin therapy. My spirits lifted after I read the evidence of common-sense reasoning that an Albarin boost to the immune system could fight invasive cancer.

My spirits instantly deflated when I found Sybil sitting alone on the edge of a half-raised rumpled bed, tears streaming down her cheeks. A breakfast tray, food untouched, sat on a portable bed table nearby. There was an open canvas sports bag spilling out lingerie and sleep shirts onto a visitor's chair. I was shocked beyond words, and I reached to take her into my arms.

"It's in my lungs," she moaned. It would not be the last time she cried, but it would be one of only a few times.

Her announcement petrified me. An agonizing shock flashed through my body. I was dumbstruck for the moment. I could not immediately grasp the enormity of her announcement.

"Oh, baby," I cried, my heart breaking for her. I felt sharp physical pain all over my body. I could hold her and kiss her, but I could not make it better.

It suddenly dawned on me that I had found her alone. I drew my head back from her shoulder.

"Where is Jayne?" I asked, thinking she was simply out of the room.

"She's gone."

"Gone home?"

She nodded gloomily.

"Was she here when the doctor told you?"

She shook her head no.

I felt so guilty to have arrived too late to be with her during this further devastating revelation. Once again, she had faced a harsh report all alone. I wish to God that I could remake that scene. Why did I not come earlier? There was no reason other than the dread of facing reality, but time would have made no difference. I should have stayed the night in order to be there, whatever the situation, but especially at the time when the doctor gave her the news.

"I'm so sorry, baby. I should have come earlier."

"It's okay," she sighed and started patting my back to comfort me. It was so like her to be a caregiver herself, in spite of her personal grief.

Then suddenly she drew back and declared angrily, "As soon as that doctor told me I had lung cancer, he had the nerve to tell me that I could go out and smoke a cigarette if I wanted to. Can you believe that?"

"What good did he think that would do? Settle your nerves?"

"Go figure," she replied.

"I'll have the nurse ask for a nicotine patch. I know you do not want to smoke anymore, but the patch will make it easier for you. Take all the help you can get. None of this is easy."

"Right now, I want a bath and shampoo. My period started, and I feel terrible."

"Well, at least I can help you with that." I was relieved to be able to do something for her.

We made our way gingerly toward the bathroom, her left arm over my shoulder and my right one around her waist. She limped into the shower stall and sat down heavily onto the chair that had been placed directly underneath the shower wand.

"I'll do this myself," she said.

I put shampoo and a bar of white bath soap within reach of her left hand. She always shampooed her curly brown hair daily and then used a blow-dryer to brush out some of her curls.

"Got it! I'll handle it from here," she declared with a dismissive hand motion.

"Okay, honey. Let's ditch that hospital garb. I'll get one of your own gowns. Meanwhile, you go ahead and soap up, and I will rinse and towel you dry. Call me when you are ready."

She called for me only after she finished the shampoo, shower, and rinse. I patted her dry with a towel, but she dressed herself. It was important to her that she do as much as possible on her own before asking for help. I would learn to allow that, sometimes to a fault, so that she would feel less crippled.

The bath did wonders for Sybil. She was suddenly more cheerful. A friendly nurse's assistant popped her head in the door to ask, "Ready for a bath?" Sybil laughed. "Too late," she said, and patted her shiny groomed locks.

When I shared the information about aloe vera treatment that I had found on the Internet, Sybil regained hope and determination for a battle against the enemy that was taking over her body.

It was mid-morning when Randy and Bill walked in together. Soon thereafter, a stream of doctors began to arrive. Thankfully, Randy was there to witness the specific plans ordered by the oncologist. My mind raced too madly with emotional turmoil to understand the facts. Truthfully, I was afraid we were going to face even more alarming information.

It was not like TV, with a group of "scrubs" gathering around Sybil's bed ready to treat her all at the same time and offering assurances of success and guaranteed recovery. Instead, they arrived one at a time, some in business suits. None of them exuded reassurance.

Dr. Edward Bert Knight, a pulmonologist specializing in treatment and management of diseases of the lungs and airways, was the first specialist to arrive. Dr. Knight was affiliated with Lung and Chest Medical Associates in Spartanburg, and he would be conducting tests of her lung tumor to determine the type of cancer Sybil was stricken with and whether it would be operable. The type of cancer found in the lung would determine whether she would be a candidate for the brain surgery. Regardless of the bodily connection, we were praying that surgery could be done to get those debilitating tumors out of Sybil's brain; for us, having a tumor in the brain was the worst of the worse. Dr. Knight explained his role in the upcoming tests and said that an anesthesiologist, whose name I did not catch, would come to talk to her as well.

All emphasis was now on lung cancer, and with that came a frightful prospect. For there is an aggressive type of inoperable lung cancer that is not confined to the lungs: small cell carcinoma, sometimes called "oat cell carcinoma" because its cells are rounded and flat, like oat grains. It has the most rapid clinical course of any type of lung cancer. Small cell lung cancer can produce an abnormal abundance of hormones, which leads to adverse secondary effects. It has a greater tendency to escape early detection, so that by the time it is diagnosed, it has already spread widely; in the majority of diagnosed patients, it has also metastasized. Metastasis had already occurred in Sybil, but the doctors had yet to determine whether the cancer in her brain was small cell carcinoma.

Meanwhile, the hospital staff made plans for the usual invasive options: radiation and chemotherapy.

Dr. Drew Monitto, a radiation oncologist affiliated with Spartanburg Radiation Oncology Associates, made an appearance to introduce himself. He was prepared to begin the radiation therapy immediately following the other procedures.

In spite of the seriousness of the situation, I could not help but notice that the neurosurgeon, Dr. Cavert McCorkle, was a tall and extremely handsome man. He was also quite charming during his introductions to each of us. He assured Sybil that he was on call to do the surgery if an operation proved possible. I was further impressed when June, a close friend of Sybil's and a resident of Spartanburg, came to visit later that day and gave an excellent report on the surgeon's reputation in the city. The following day, Dr. McCorkle further endeared himself to me when he flatteringly mistook me for my daughter as I greeted him upon his arrival. I was also touched that he was making daily contact with Sybil and monitoring the results of the necessary tests. His sincerity and attentiveness displayed a compassion that I did not find in his oncologist colleague, Dr. Corso. The oncologist would stride hurriedly into the room, speak brusquely, and take his leave. His cool professional approach certainly allowed him to maintain an emotional distance from his patients, and perhaps that was the reason he needed to maintain an aloof image.

There was a continuous stream of other medical personnel garbed in sick green jackets and hairnets. These included the anesthesiologist who administered anesthesia during the prearranged lung tests and the lab technician who brought a cart of tubes, one labeled with Sybil's name, for blood samples. The nurses who came in periodically were dressed in bright flowered smocks. I thought this dress code was sad. I remembered the white starched caps and uniforms nurses once wore. There was reassurance in that professional appearance, and their dress commanded a certain respect. It was different with these street colors and flowered blouses. Nevertheless, no matter how they were clad, all the hospital personnel were ominous to me.

Thus began our journey into a world that was foreign and terrifying to our entire family. The urgency of Sybil's earth-shattering diagnosis did not allow us the luxury of taking time to reflect on decisions. The choices were slim to almost none.

While the activity swirled around us at the hospital, Randy armed himself, via telephone calls, with all the information he could gather on the Albarin treatment. Joseph DiStefano, the practitioner who ran the Florida clinic, welcomed his calls and was eager to answer all of his questions. DiStefano told him that the aloe vera treatment treats all types of cancer, but there is a greater chance that it would be more effective if the cancer began in the lungs and went to the brain later, as Sybil's did, because of something to do with breaking a blood barrier in the neck going upward to the brain. Judging by Randy's reports, the treatment in Florida seemed as if it would be very beneficial for Sybil. DiStefano would not say "cure," but he did say that he had had a lot of success treating cancer with Albarin. Pat talked with Randy daily, calling from wherever in the world his Delta flights took him. He began to call the hospital as well, to ask about Sybil. He was quite concerned about her and encouraged us to consider the Albarin therapy.

But first we had to wait and see whether the cancer in her brain was operable. As we faced that dilemma, I continued to hope that surgery would be possible and that the tumors could be removed from Sybil's brain. The tumors in her brain were responsible for the numbness in her leg and arm. Although the cancer began in her lungs, that seemed secondary to the more destructive cancer in her head. Further lung testing was necessary before they could consider brain surgery.

Dr. Corso informed us that if it were small cell carcinoma, it would be inoperable. Dr. Knight was going to perform a lung biopsy to obtain a tissue sample for culture. Dr. McCorkle was standing by with possible surgery appointment times in case it turned out to be non-small cell and allowed a surgical solution. Dr. Menitto prepared for radiation treatment in any event.

We could do nothing more than wait, pray, and hope.

The Word Spread

Sybil's friends and family rally around

We waited anxiously for two days to get an answer from Dr. Knight, and it was a non-answer. The first test was inconclusive, which I hoped was a good sign. Immediately upon hearing the results, Dr. Knight made plans to perform another biopsy. This procedure involved making a small opening in her back and thus required general anesthesia. The test was scheduled to take place Friday morning in the hospital operating room.

Meanwhile, word of Sybil's tragedy spread swiftly in Forest City, the small North Carolina town that our family had called home for over thirty years. Forest City, population approximately seven thousand, was a close-knit community during Sybil's youth, and she had played a big part in the friendly village atmosphere, interacting with all the residents as if they were family. She kept those relationships alive into adulthood.

Now, many years later, in Spartanburg, South Carolina, a steady stream of friends strode into her private hospital space while we waited for the final word on her diagnosis and treatment options. Calls came from Colorado, Ohio, Florida, and elsewhere. Flowers filled the shelf space, and cards created a bright new wall decor in the sterile room. There were former classmates, family members, neighbors old and new, co-workers, and her pastor. All were stunned by the seriousness of her condition.

Bill said, "She touched a lot of people, and she pulled a community together. She really did."

Bill's mother, Lib, and his sister-in-law, Lynn, drove a hundred miles from Lincolnton, North Carolina, to the hospital. Lib expressed concern about her plans to go on a vacation to central Florida the following week. She was reluctant to leave North Carolina during this unexpected crisis. Sybil and I exchanged knowing glances but did not tell Lib about our research and the real possibility that we, too, might be leaving for Florida if circumstances continued to worsen in this oncology unit. Each discouraging diagnosis made Joe DiStefano's St. Petersburg clinic a more viable and promising option. We kept our silence on that subject, but both Sybil and I insisted that Lib continue with her planned trip.

The bedside telephone rang constantly with queries from other friends and family members who could not come in person. In fact, there were so many calls that it became necessary to ask a few of our friends to relay information to others. We contacted the designated ones with updates so that they could pass it along. It was a good plan that helped maintain a quieter atmosphere in the room.

On the evening before the scheduled surgical biopsy, Sybil and I were both delighted when we glimpsed the soles of a man's shoes and the front of a wheelchair gliding carefully through the door. We knew it had to be her beloved friend, Tommy Hicks. Tommy's attendant, Johnny Carson, wheeled in Sybil's classmate and lifelong pal. Tommy, owner and publisher of *The Amazin' Shopper*, a Rutherford County newspaper, led a small convoy of former classmates: Danny Philbeck, vice president of enrollment at Spartanburg Methodist College, David Smith, financial advisor with Edward Jones, and Burwell Byers, co-owner and manager of North State Gas in Forest City. These were handsome, genuinely devoted young men who had remained steadfastly loyal to Sybil for over thirty years. It was wonderful to see them! Their compassion touched my heart.

The old gang launched into a litany of memories, rolling gaily from their lips one after another. "Do you remember when ——?" They talked about football, baseball, cheerleading, prom, who had dated whom, graffiti on the water tank, and the time Mr. Morris, the principal, caught Sybil sitting in the parking lot with Mike Nanney during classes.

Their jolly chatter thrilled Sybil. The happy picture included none of the underlying thoughts about the gravity of Sybil's physical condition. She was radiant and beautiful. Her face beaming brightly above a stunning red sleep shirt, her dark eyes shining with joy. I was so happy for her that special evening.

The evening was interrupted when young Dr. Corso rushed in the door with his usual demeanor and jaunty air. But the oncologist's attitude suddenly changed to uncertainty when he found himself thrust into a room full of Sybil's young male supporters. The unexpected merriment seemed to astonish him. And Sybil's cheerfulness disarmed him after he had made his way uncomfortably through the assemblage of visitors to her bedside.

"How … uh … how are you doing?" He stuttered slightly in an attempt to regain his cool professional manner.

Sybil's eyes glistened as she swept her left arm around to take in the young men in the room. She was smiling a broad, happy smile. "How do you think I'm doing?" The positive effect her visitors had on her was obvious.

The young doctor was made visibly uncomfortable by the unexpected gaiety of his patient. Obviously, medical school had not prepared him for this type of attitude. He quickly reminded her of the scheduled procedure for the next day, and made an abrupt exit. He would come to discover more about her self-control in a few days.

The ring of the telephone, which I hastily answered, did not interrupt the chatter in the room. It was Bill. When he heard our background noise, he asked, laughingly, "What's going on there?"

I backed away from the group and turned my head so that I could hear him over the jolly banter in the room. There was loud background noise on his end of the line also.

"We've got a half dozen of Sybil's old boyfriends visiting, including Tommy Hicks," I told him. "And what kind of party are you having?"

Still laughing, he replied, "Kenny Hankinson stopped by the shop with a bottle of Jack Daniels, so the guys and I are just …"

"Just?"

"Just hangin' out," he finished.

"Well, whatever. Sounds like you are having a fun evening. And for the moment, so is Sybil." Friends at both places were offering as much support and cheer as they knew how.

Bill did not want to interrupt the visit with her friends by asking to speak with her. "Tell Sybil that I'll be at the hospital before her biopsy in the morning."

The clatter in the room shifted to plans about their upcoming class reunion and the party get-togethers that they would enjoy beforehand. She was always excited about plans for their periodic reunions. As senior class secretary, Sybil was heavily involved in the organization and planning of each one. She always shared the plans and schedules with me, bubbling with thoughts of seeing everyone again. The reunion committee, which enjoyed the planning as much or more than the actual reunions, usually gathered at Tommy's house, a beautiful and spacious home built to accommodate his wheelchair activities. Tommy's porch is a chair path that wraps around the entire house. The home and pond sit privately in the middle of a large grassy field, giving them a perfect spot to have fun evenings during the brainstorming for the big celebration of their high school days.

Sybil's spirits were enormously uplifted during the stimulating reminiscent trail of memories with her friends. In addition, envisioning the upcoming reunion festivities excited her. Her dear friends had succeeded in their drop-in mission to cheer and support her. That evening was like a brief recess, a bittersweet highlight tucked among the bad tidings that now flooded her days.

I am truly grateful to those young men who came to let her know how much they cared for her. Tommy later remembered the evening at the hospital, "Yes, it was a great night for us all. I hope Sybil knew how much we loved her. Even in that situation Sybil and I could tease each other, and I'll never forget how beautiful she was that night in her hot red gown."

We both felt the warmth of the evening when I tucked her in with a good-night kiss before I pulled down the Murphy bed to sleep beside her.

On Friday morning, January 19, I felt a sense of loss as I watched a young orderly deftly slide Sybil from her hospital bed onto a gurney that would take her to another part of the hospital. *What are we doing here? We do not belong in this place,* I was thinking. It was time again to determine what type cancer she had and to learn whether the operation would be possible. Dr. McCorkle was standing by, ready to do the surgery on Monday if need be.

"I'll make the phone calls and join you when I finish," I told Sybil as the bed rolled past me. I would report to our telephone network even though the only news I had to relay was that we would have no further information until Monday. This report would at least keep the phone lines clear over the weekend.

Bill walked alongside her as they moved into the corridor. I felt a chill as I stood alone in the deserted sterile room. It took a few moments for me to focus on the situation at hand. A review of the whole situation from my perspective brought to light the realization that I had better take some action. There was no question about staying at my daughter's side for the duration, whether that meant surgery or an alternative clinic. Looking realistically at the total picture, I saw that it was necessary that I give up my part-time job.

A no-brainer demands immediate attention. My phone card was on the night table beside the telephone. I picked it up to call Billy Joe. After giving him the day's update about Sybil, I said, "BJ,

I have never in my life quit a job without advance notice, but I have no choice right now. I can't possibly go back to work until Sybil is well, and I have no idea how long that will be."

"I understand, Iris, but you don't have to quit. Just take all the time off that you need," he said compassionately.

"I appreciate that, BJ, but I know already that it is going to take a long time for her to recover, and I simply cannot ask you to wait. It wouldn't be fair to you."

He repeated, "But you don't need to quit. I understand your situation, and I can wait."

"Billy Joe, we are strongly considering taking her to Florida for treatment. You'll need some help before I get back."

"You still don't have to quit."

"I know you understand, and I really appreciate it. It's been such a pleasure working with you, and I really would like to come back, but right now it doesn't seem likely that I can." His understanding touched me. It was very kind of him to keep my job open. Nevertheless, I did not want to inconvenience him for an undetermined time.

Although Billy Joe did not accept my resignation, I did in my own mind, if only so I would not feel guilty about being away.

That task behind me, I made the calls to our assigned messengers to pass today's word around before I left the room to find Sybil and Bill.

The oncology building was an addition to the older traditional hospital. The buildings were connected by a conglomeration of halls. I kept losing my way in the maze of confusing angles and turns. When I stopped to ask, I still took wrong turns. I was nearly in tears when I finally found the couple. By that time, the procedure was over and Sybil was already beginning to wake up.

"How do you feel?" I asked.

When she turned toward me to answer, she winced, "Oh," she cried out, "my back." It startled her to hit a sore spot.

"It hurts where the incision was made?"

She nodded. "Not much. I just didn't remember where the needle went in."

Bill and I went back to the hospital room with Sybil. Since we would not be able to learn anything over the weekend, there was no need for Sybil to stay in the hospital until the results came in.

"Let's check out of this hotel," I told them," there is too much room service, but no wine."

"Amen!" Sybil laughed.

"I'll go downstairs to check you out while you get ready, Sybil. The two of you can meet me down in the lobby."

Dr. Corso promised that he would telephone her with the results as soon as he found out.

We drove back to Forest City hoping to spend a quiet weekend waiting for the results. Part of the plan backfired, however, when our telephone network excitedly broadcast that she would be home for a couple days. Sybil's well-meaning friends flocked to see her, and though she was pleased to see them, it was physically painful and mentally exhausting. There were none of the restrictions on visiting hours that a hospital enforces. The tiring weekend would influence future homecoming rules.

However, there was one good thing to the flurry of activity during the break from the medical facility: the commotion took some attention away from the stressful thoughts about upcoming results of the lung biopsy.

When I went to join Sybil and Bill at their home for another trip to the oncology unit on Monday morning, I had not yet heard news of the medical analysis of the lung biopsy. I rang the doorbell and called out when I opened the louvered glass door and walked through the sunroom. Sybil's welcoming response drew me into the kitchen's dining area, where I found her perched at the end of the kitchen bar, gazing into a mirror that was propped on the counter beside a small basket of makeup paraphernalia. She had a mascara wand in her hand and a frown on her face. She paused in her cosmetic application to exchange a loving hug with me. She then proceeded to roll color on her long eyelashes. I noticed that she was holding her right hand with her good left one to direct the application. Her short brunette curls were smooth and shiny. Her eyelashes were a final addition to a picture of a lovely girl who was not happy now.

"Good morning," I said lightly.

"It happened again," she said sorrowfully, while looking into the small round mirror.

"What happened again?"

She pointed to her mouth with the eyelash stick, "Numb again."

That familiar chilling shock spread through my being again. "When?"

"Just now, a few minutes ago."

Then she said, abruptly, "Dr. Corso didn't call me this morning. A person from radiology called to inform me that I have an appointment there this morning at nine o'clock."

"What?' I asked bewildered, "Why?"

The sudden radiation appointment, however, was an explanation in itself. It was somberly apparent that even though Dr. McCorkle had set aside an appointment for her, she would not be having surgery. It also indicated, to our disappointment, that surgery was no longer a promising option.

We immediately took our angry frustration out on Dr. Corso, who had not called personally as he had promised. He had shown blatant disrespect and a lack of compassion for Sybil.

"The very least he could have done was to call you himself," I complained bitterly. The call that she received simply informed her of a scheduled appointment without further explanation. Of course, we guessed the reasoning without knowing the extent of it, but it was the doctor's duty to make the call.

"We're not going to keep that appointment," Bill declared firmly. "We're going to have a meeting with Dr. Corso to find out what all the facts are." He was pacing nervously. They had decided before my arrival that we would go to Spartanburg to confront the doctor. Sybil was not going to allow someone to make decisions for her without her approval.

I drove alone to the hospital, prepared to stay overnight with my daughter if she decided to stay. I tried to think positively and prayed for favorable news. I allowed myself to hope that radiation could kill the tumors in her brain. (That was not logical, however. Radiation sufficient to kill the cancer cells was bound to kill her good brain cells as well.)

I started a prayer that became my daily ritual in the mornings and at bedtime. "Dear God, please clear, heal, and cure her." I believed God would heal her. All my life, I found myself blessed with answered prayers. I saw no reason why this one could not be answered as well. Sybil, after all, was someone who could make a positive difference in the world around her.

I joined the couple in the parking lot, and the three of us went directly to Dr. Corso's office. "We want to talk with Dr. Corso," Bill stated determinedly.

The nurse was hesitant. Of course, she knew who we were and that we had not kept the appointment that Dr. Corso had prearranged with radiology. "He is seeing patients now. He just started his rounds. I don't know whether he can see you." She was obviously trying to discourage us, because we were insisting on a consultation without an appointment. "He has other appointments scheduled this morning."

"Tell him that we are here. We'll wait," Bill told her resolutely.

When she saw our determination, she reluctantly escorted us directly into his office, bypassing the waiting room where other patients were waiting for their appointments. She pulled a chair from one side of the room to make seating for three, putting the extra chair between two upholstered chairs. Sybil sat in the center chair.

"I'll tell the doctor that you are waiting," she said as she left the room. She allowed us privacy by closing the door softly behind her.

We started talking excitedly about the treatment center in

Florida. By now, we had gathered enough information from Pat, Randy, and some of Joe DiStefano's current patients to feel positive about the therapy. I became even more convinced as they told me some of the testimonials they had heard. It offered hope.

We had a long wait, and eventually we fell silent, weary and anxious for the doctor to hurry. I wondered if he was deliberately delaying the encounter because we had disrupted his orders for radiation. When Dr. Corso at last strode in, he had an emotionless expression on his face.

"What's going on, Doctor?" Bill asked.

He did not answer immediately. He grasped the back of his desk chair and swirled it around toward Sybil. Then he sat down abruptly and bent forward to face her. Without warning he blurted out a curt, shocking announcement.

"The tumor is small cell carcinoma and inoperable."

We were speechless. He reached for a white legal pad on his desk, took a pen from his jacket pocket, and proceeded to coolly sketch illustrations and write. Then looked and pointed at the sketches as he spoke brusquely.

"You have a large tumor on the left side and a smaller one on the right. We will start you on radiation for the large lesion immediately. Two continuous weeks." He wrote the number and added more. "One week of rest between the two-week series until it shrinks, and then a strict regime of chemotherapy." Then suddenly, in the same blunt tone, he declared, "With no treatment, you will die within three months."

Words cannot define the searing shockwaves that spread throughout my body. I refused to accept that dreadful and unexpected declaration. I wanted to scream, to escape. This man was sentencing Sybil to death with his absolute proclamation. My body went numb. I could not move. I could not think clearly. I did not think I heard correctly. *His harsh words could not be true.*

Bill, too, was speechless, but Sybil bravely found her voice. "And with treatment, how long?" Her voice was clear but trembling.

"Oh … uh, given your age and healthy condition, you should

live longer with radiation and chemotherapy, maybe even as much as a year," he answered, casually and indifferently.

My mind was racing wildly. I was thinking about the Albarin treatment.

"And what about alternative treatments?" I did not know what to ask that would do anything to render his verdict wrong or change it.

He answered offhandedly. "I have no objection to you trying something alternative during the break between radiation treatments. And you are welcome to get a second opinion from another oncologist."

The doctor expected Sybil to follow his orders. "While you are here, you will reschedule the radiation treatment for tomorrow." Confident that Sybil would follow his instruction, he dismissed us and directed his nurse to show Sybil the way to the radiology department.

There was nothing but doom in his pronouncement. Doom is not something our family is accustomed to accepting. This was no exception. The news was dreadful, and the bearer of the news offered no compassion. In this case, I was willing to "shoot the messenger."

While the nurse gave Sybil directions to radiology, I asked Bill, "Will you call Randy? I'll go with Sybil."

"Yeah, I'll call Randy," Bill promised and reached for his cell phone.

As Sybil and I walked away from the nurse in the direction she had indicated, Sybil told me emphatically, "I will never come back to this place."

"Okay," I said wryly, "but security will probably stop us if we don't schedule you again. You broke one appointment, and you can make and break another. It'll serve them right after the way they treated you today."

She grinned as we walked casually up to the receptionist desk at radiology where an appointment card was already prepared.

The receptionist stated the hour as she handed the card across to Sybil. "Nine o'clock tomorrow morning."

Sybil murmured a weak thank you, and we walked away to the first outside door.

Bill was waiting for us. "Randy is leaving now to come to Forest City."

Sybil's refusal to accept Dr. Corso's terrible proposal left only one avenue open to us. The alternate choice would have to be the alternative approach. So, leaving the gloom and doom of the hospital, we readied ourselves for the little-known experiment, Albarin.

She Chose Hope

Sybil and I board a flight toward a chance for life

The Palmetto Oncology Clinic doors that closed behind us turned off the mental alarm that Dr. Corso set off. We walked away from that prison of hopelessness with immense relief and a sense of freedom. Sybil would not come back here. She would never be locked away to be eaten and burned alive by chemicals that kill both cancerous and healthy cells.

Sybil, Bill, and I breathed in the refreshing crisp air. With that load lifted from our minds, we strode to our cars with renewed hope. I followed them to their home, confident that Sybil was prepared and determined to go forward with a plan to save her life. We would travel this path together and face any obstacles with resolute optimism.

The question that Bill and Sybil discussed on their way home was not why they should try the Albarin treatment but why not. The only practical recourse seemed to be Joe DiStefano's clinical trial. Should that therapy happen to fail, the disease would destroy her body, not cell-killing chemicals. The aloe treatment is safe, harmless, and hopeful. It would not harm.

Now that all hope was gone for anything good to come from the Spartanburg hospital, Sybil made up her mind to try the promising Albarin therapy. She looked forward to enjoying

Florida's warm weather and the warm welcome that Joe and his staff had offered thus far.

Sybil's pastor, David Hobson, best described the courage that led to her conclusion. Pastor Hobson is a large man, with brown hair and matching beard beautifully highlighted with silver, a pleasant smile, and a twinkle in his eye. I think he is a teddy bear with a big heart, kind and loving. He speaks slowly and deliberately, each word full of easily understood meaning and eloquently delivered. A listener wants to grasp his every word as I did when he talked to me about Sybil's determination to fight the cancer.

"Spartanburg," he said, "was a very cold and calculated place that said, 'Well, you know, these are your chances.' But that's not how she lived her life, so that's not how she wanted to face her death, if that was what was in store for her. That is certainly not how she wanted to fight the cancer. She certainly did not want to say, 'Well, I'll just let the cancer wash me away.' She said, 'No, if it takes me, it will have to fight every step of the way. It will have to fight me until it can't fight anymore or until I can't. And while I'm doing this battle, it won't be a battle going on grim, bitter, or even focused on myself. Instead, it will be a battle waged with love, optimism, and openness to other's needs. That's how I'll fight this battle.'

"It was clear from her spirit, from the time we learned of her cancer and began the process with her, that she was a person who faced what she had in front of her with a very realistic perspective. She faced the challenge. She faced it not only with courage but also with optimism. She faced it in such a way that people around her were encouraged. Generally, that's what works best in a family that's fighting cancer. If the patient is easily discouraged, then the family is almost made powerless. But her courage and her willingness to face this and to attempt this challenge with all her being was powerful. She was going to handle this and deal with this. She wasn't just going to let it wash her away.

"There was constancy in her from the first time that I went down to Spartanburg until the day we got the results. We dealt with the news that the cancer was malignant and so powerful that there was no optimism whatsoever on the part of the people in Spartanburg. But rather than just lie down and take it, she said, 'I'm going to find an option. I'm going to look at different options. I am not going to take it lying down.' And she took that option and worked it as hard and as long and as far as she could."

The pastor well understood Bill and Sybil's resolution to opt for a new trial procedure.

Randy arrived in Forest City shortly after we returned from Spartanburg, in spite of driving twice the distance. Sybil, Bill, and I were waiting restlessly for him in their kitchen. He gave us each a loving hug, then perched himself on a barstool at the kitchen counter to chart our course. He paused only now and then to take a sip or two from his water bottle. Randy was obviously anxious and talked rapidly, as he always does when he is excited.

"I've already talked with Joe, talked to him on the way down here. He encouraged me to bring you to St. Petersburg," he said to Sybil. "He can start treatment right away, starting tomorrow, if we can be there. He is not allowed to say that he can cure you, but he could say that he has had a lot of success in treating cancer. One thing he stated firmly is, 'She's got small-cell carcinoma. It's a fast-growing cancer. You're welcome to come here, but if you do not bring her here, get treatment somewhere.' That's the kind of person he is, really caring about anyone who needs help."

Randy's excitement was contagious. We put the somber Spartanburg ordeal out of our mind and replaced it with lighthearted hopefulness. Our attitude became positive and optimistic as our aspirations and determination shifted toward a new and promising treatment. We sprang into action.

Bill said, "Kenny Hankinson will fly you down. He told me he can have a plane up in the air anytime."

Randy said, "I'll drive your car down, Sybil. You and Mom can fly with Kenny." (There was no discussion about whether I would be going. It was simply assumed, and rightly so.) "I'll take the treatments with you. I've been planning to, for maintenance anyway. Bill, you call Kenny, and I'll call Joe's office and see if they can recommend a place for us to stay in St. Petersburg." Randy directed us as he hastily made plans and reached for a portable telephone that lay on the counter.

We were thankful that my son took charge of the sudden arrangements. The morning's experience in the oncology clinic had mentally drained the three of us.

Joe's receptionist, Nancy, answered his call. They had already become phone friends during Randy's recent daily calls to the clinic. She recommended Grant Motel, a place that some of their patients had stayed during treatments, and gave him the address and telephone number.

He immediately called the motel to make arrangements. They assured Randy that there was a vacancy. While making the reservations, he looked at us with a grin. He was amused by the motel clerk's British accent.

Bill placed a call to KCH Service, the manufacturing company Kenny owns, but Kenny was not in. I was afraid that we might not find Kenny before the day was out. Kenny was personally involved in many community affairs and was often out of town on business. He could be anywhere. While Bill told the KCH secretary to have him call right away, I brushed aside that worry.

"I'll go home and pack," I said, suddenly cheered by promise to our prayers. Joe DiStefano, I thought, had shown compassion for my daughter sight unseen. How grateful I was! Flight or not, we would be going to Florida. I prepared myself for the long drive down in case Kenny could not be found.

On my way home, I called my grandson, Chad. He was my dependable house-sitter. The arrangement worked well for both of us. At that time, he was a young single man; he enjoyed being on his own during my travels, and I felt secure about my home while away. He was glad to be of help during this crisis. I only needed to worry about what baggage I would carry for this trip of unknown duration. It seemed that Sybil would have at least thirty treatments. So maybe we would stay two months, possibly more.

I rushed into the house and upstairs to get my carry-on bag from the closet. It already contained some overnight essentials (toothbrush, toothpaste, shampoo, other hair products, basic makeup, etc.). That was a good thing right then, because I found myself simply staring into the clothes closet without seeing individual garments. I could not concentrate. A loud ring from the telephone jarred me back to reality.

"Kenny will be ready to take off for Florida at four o'clock. You can meet us at the airport and leave your car there. I'll have Chad pick it up later."

I looked at my wristwatch. It was three o'clock. "I'll be there!"

I set the phone back on its cradle and spoke to myself out loud. "Okay, Iris, get with the program!" A few warm slacks and tops, hangers of basic black and brown pants, some blouses and sweaters. I simply took everything from the lingerie drawers and hurriedly stuffed everything into a suitcase. I could worry about wrinkles later.

What the heck, I thought. *This is not important. If I only have the clothes on my back, I can wash them as needed.*

Meanwhile, Bill was helping Sybil do the same thing. She loved to wear her sweats, so they packed several of them. Neither of us gave much thought to the warmer Florida weather. Here in western North Carolina, it is cold in January. Nevertheless, we just wanted to get to the clinic as soon as possible. Other matters could take care of themselves one way or another.

I thought about collecting something to snack on during the flight. There had been too much activity for us to eat breakfast or lunch. I found cheese, crackers, water, and a bit of Chardonnay. I was feeling light-hearted about escaping the ten-day nightmare we had just endured. Sybil's disease would be with us, but we were going to a place where we expected the cancer would be destroyed.

Sybil asked me to bring a tape recorder so that she could record this experience. I reached for one of the two that were on my office bookshelf and opened a drawer to get extra batteries and blank cassettes. Then I took a deep breath and mentally reviewed what I had for the trip. I put the tape paraphernalia into a shopping bag along with the snacks and carried it in one hand while I pulled the carry-on to the car. Then I went back into the house to collect my purse and shut off the thermostat and computer. If there was anything else, Chad could take care of it when he came he came to house-sit. I did not have the time to follow my usual instincts and double-check everything.

My heart beat rapidly as I locked the door and rushed to the car. Glancing quickly at my watch, I found that there was barely enough time to go by the ATM on East Main Street on my way to the airport. I drove through the quiet downtown of Forest City, where carefully tended trees, shrubbery, and multicolored pansies beautifully separated the right and left lanes of traffic. As I passed Smith's drugstore, I pictured the local characters who habitually gather at the old-fashioned soda fountain, men's hands fidgeting with aged white crackled coffee mugs, unaware of our family's personal crisis. They are a consistent group, slowly rotating from high school to grave, and they are there practically every weekday morning except the week of the Fourth of July, when they all go to Myrtle Beach. On the other side of the street, another group gathers at Ron and Eddy's restaurant; different characters, same scene.

Some of these regulars once frequented a town restaurant that is no longer in existence, Cracker Barrel. Sybil was a part-time server at Cracker Barrel during her high school years, cheerfully greeting diners with her bright smile and brilliant sense of humor. She was fond of all the regulars, those now divided between the drugstore and Ron & Eddy's café. I was sure they still remembered her over twenty years later. She would smile brightly and flip her coffee decanter just so, tilt it once, and fill the cup without spilling a drop. I still marvel at her ability to pour one spurt of liquid out of a pitcher and have it be just the right amount for the cup or glass. It is a little thing, I know, but the little things stab my heart the most when I remember her. I have a steel wall built to protect me from the big things, but small memories sneak through the cracks to bring hurt to my heart and tears to my eyes.

Sybil's health report would reach their ears by the next day, I realized. Her condition would become the breakfast club's foremost topic of the day for many weeks to come. They would remember her beauty and her friendly personality.

On the left is a beautiful water fountain that showers a crystal dome of water spray within a circle of a black lacy iron fence. The fountain is a recurring target for soapsuds tossed carelessly by young fun loving teens looking for a mischievous thrill.

I now felt more relaxed than I had since the night Sybil told me of the first scheduled MRI. I felt very good about this trip. It was exciting to know that hope lay ahead for us.

I passed the building that once housed Cracker Barrel and had since been converted into the largest used car dealership in the county. A couple blocks beyond was the building that used to be Cool Springs Middle School, where Sybil first became a cheerleader. And she never stopped being a cheerleader. She was still cheering on those same classmates, in spite of her illness, as well as cheering on all her family and friends.

A fog of memories faded in and out during my drive. I passed the "Welcome to Forest City" sign on Main Street and turned onto Hudlow Road, a five-mile two-lane country road that leads to Highway 64. Soon I was turning onto Airport Road.

On reaching the airport parking lot, flanked by small one-story buildings, I watched Bill help Sybil out of their four-door Buick sedan. Straight ahead, on the other side of a chain link fence, two men were busy prepping a sleek white Cessna 340, striped with blue and numbered N5070C.

As we strolled toward the tarmac at Sybil's pace, Kenny stepped forward and greeted us politely, and then he introduced his co-pilot, George Ronan, who was also the airport manager. A good-looking pair, I observed, and apparently very efficient. They quietly and quickly relieved us of our carry-on bags. Kenny tossed them nonchalantly onto the rear bench seat of the aircraft before assisting us aboard.

Sybil and I sat facing each other in single seats beside the window. We grinned at each other and giggled excitedly about flying away to a new life. Our hearts overflowed with the delight of hope, and our sparkling eyes mirrored that feeling. This was yet another star in the crown of adventures that we had shared over the years. We loved to travel together.

Our accommodating pilots bent forward as they silently entered through the rear door and filed past us to the cockpit. Kenny and George easily settled into their pilot seats. It was evident that they were regular flying companions. They were laid back, as if this was an ordinary flight. But they both knew it was more than just an ordinary flight plan. This was a mission. Before he took the controls, Kenny turned around, leaned over toward us, and handed me a roll of folded green bills.

"Tommy Hicks sent this to you," he said kindly.

"Thank you," I said, surprised. And then I turned back toward Sybil. "Look, Sybil." I passed her the money. "From Tommy, bless his heart." Sybil's dear friend Tommy and their mutual friends and former classmates simply wanted to help her, doing so without fanfare.

She flashed a bright smile. "Oh, he shouldn't have done that! That is so sweet." She handed the money back to me. "Here, you take care of it."

Kenny and George were now engaged in takeoff procedures. We glided up without a ripple and rose above the open landscape of winter's straw-colored grass, naked trees, and evergreens divided by the tiny lines of roads. The smooth takeoff and their relaxed manner set us at ease. We settled into a comfortable, easy conversation.

"Remember your first flight?" I asked Sybil, with a smile. She had an early fear of flying. For her first experience, Linda, our employee, and I accompanied Sybil on a short hop to Atlanta.

She nodded and laughed. "Yes, I do. A couple of Bloody Marys, and I was high enough to fly."

"Linda and I didn't let you drink alone."

"That's what friends are for."

"Remember how I kept trying to get Linda to shut up? The minute we buckled our seat belts, she started a running commentary of 'close call' airplane episodes. A tire blowout, a near miss, an emergency landing, and stuff like that. There we were, deliberately attempting to help you fly without fear, and she was pumping us with frightful scenarios. I did not want to make an issue out of it, so I kept giving her dirty looks behind your back, whenever I could catch her eye. She just laughed and ignored me. She enjoyed teasing you."

"She made you more nervous than me. I was not paying any attention. I was trying to do the deep breathing you told me to do." Sybil smiled. She had also chewed gum like crazy as a substitute for cigarettes. "The entire trip was a blast."

"And remember the van driver looking for the big chicken?"

"The 'beeg cheeken,'" Sybil laughingly imitated the Latino driver from our hotel as she remembered the incident. The young immigrant was driving us in the hotel van to a special restaurant recommended by the concierge. He did not know the location, and so he called the hotel to ask directions. "The beeg cheeken?" we heard him say. Sybil and Linda giggled in the double seat directly behind the driver. "Si," he replied confidently, and then he began speeding through the city streets, making turns along the way. Soon he slowed and began turning his head right and left, looking absolutely confused. Dumbfounded, he rang up his dispatcher again. "Si, the beeg cheeken," he confirmed once again when he heard directions. He then turned toward us to reassure us that the restaurant "is beside the beeg cheeken." We burst into laughter. Someone said, "Let's get going to the 'beeg cheeken.'" When the van finally stopped beside Kentucky Fried Chicken but at the wrong restaurant, we just threw up our hands and left him in the vehicle to find his way back to the hotel. It no longer mattered what we ate; we were having a jolly time anyway.

After our meal, a different driver came to pick us up from the restaurant. When we entered the van, evangelistic rhetoric was blasting from the radio.

"And after the 'beeg cheeken' there was the sermon. Amen!" Sybil said, still laughing as she recalled the second jaunt of that evening.

We had seated ourselves in the hotel van, but our driver barely acknowledged us because he was engrossed in the evangelist's preaching. Suddenly the man exclaimed loudly, "Amen!" in response to the broadcasting reverend.

"Amen," Sybil repeated after him, and Linda followed with a louder "Amen!" They giggled, and I shushed them, fearing that the man would be insulted. Meanwhile, I was trying to suppress laughter myself. He seemed, or at least pretended, to be oblivious to our tittering. He unexpectedly let out another loud "Amen!" And it was immediately echoed by Sybil and Linda, accompanied, of course, by more snickering. The trio's chorus of amens continued throughout the return drive. I stopped trying to stifle their fun and joined them with laughter.

"And then the lesbians tried to pick up Linda," Sybil recalled.

"They were really taken with her and wanted to take her home with them."

"Everything was funny that weekend," Sybil said, now immersed in the memories. "Those girls were serious about their offer to Linda."

"And, fortunately, you haven't been afraid of flying since that hilarious weekend."

"I haven't. I am glad I got over the fear. After that first trip, I had that fun trip with Jayne to Las Vegas, another one with you, and more," she recalled.

She returned to the present. "And this is one plane ride that I consider a blessing," she said excitedly.

"I dub this an Angel Flight. We are floating on the wings of two saviors who are kind enough to take us up to heavenly skies for a journey to the great physician, Dr. Joe," I said.

"We need to drink to that," Sybil proposed.

"Good idea," I agreed and reached for our goody bag. I poured our wine, and we munched on cheese and crackers. George and Kenny had water and sandwiches in their cooler.

We stopped talking while we ate and simply enjoyed the glorious experience of winging through the downy white clouds on a blanket of the most beautiful blue I have ever witnessed. Everything was brighter than normal.

The pilots quietly communicated in their cockpit compartment, but then Kenny turned around to show us a photograph of his lovely daughter, Olivia. His pride in her was obvious. We admired Olivia, a little girl with Kenny's profile. Then Sybil passed a picture of her new granddaughter, Hannah, to Kenny and George for their compliments.

As evening fell, the smooth flight suddenly became a grand one! A wondrous orange sphere split the soft billowing clouds in layers between the white and blue. The spectacular display of heavenly colors was awesome! We sensed a heavenly embrace as we floated through the most glorious sunset any of us had ever seen.

We watched in awe, rendered mute in the midst of the spectacular display around us. We could not verbally express our feelings during the breathtaking phenomenon, which gradually faded and merged into a fully dark sky. For a short period, we found ourselves cloaked in the darkness, a warm protective shelter from the real world far below.

Kenny's voice broke through the quiet when he directed George's attention to a landing strip amid twinkling city lights that grew brighter and more colorful on our approach. "Is that it?" he asked.

Sybil and I, roused from our hypnotic trance, observed the pilots. They were searching the lighted city for the St. Petersburg–Clearwater landing strip.

"Over there," I heard one of them say.

"They can't find the airport," Sybil said.

"I don't see one either," I said as I peered through the darkness to a nest of city lights below, "but what do I know?"

"Mom, it's not your problem. You are not the pilot."

We laughed. "And that's a good thing."

Then Kenny indicated an opening he supposed might be the site they sought. "Is that it?"

"Yes, there it is."

We started to descend smoothly. I waited for a bump, but it did not come. We landed on the runway with such ease that I did not sense the landing and only realized we had landed when we were no longer moving.

Without a word, the pilots rose from their seats and scurried past us, heads down, toward the exit. We watched them stride quickly across the shadowy landing strip toward a rather dark building that seemed to be one hundred feet or more away.

"I wonder where they will get a car?" I assumed that a car rental would be in a different place than this small airport building in front of us. We settled back for a wait, and I gauged the distance Sybil would have to walk to the building. However, there was no wait, for suddenly a dark four-door sedan sped toward the aircraft and braked to a stop only a few feet away.

Sybil grinned appreciatively. "Our limo has arrived."

I was so thankful that they brought the vehicle all the way to the airplane. "Wow, I'm impressed."

Kenny crawled inside the plane to retrieve our luggage, and I reached toward Sybil to help her out of her seat. The men then stood on either side of the exit to steady her as she gingerly maneuvered down the steps and made her way to the ground. Stairs were now becoming difficult for her to manage.

Sybil and I situated ourselves in the back seat of the borrowed car. George opened a street map of St. Petersburg that he had picked up in the airport and began directing Kenny toward Grant

Motel on 9046 Fourth Street. I paid little attention to the route and had no idea where we were or where we should be going.

I made small talk with Sybil along the way, promising that we would soon be dining and dancing at some of the hotels and restaurants we were passing. In spite of Dr. Corso's ominous warning, it was my firm belief that Sybil came to St. Petersburg for the cure that would rid her of cancer.

We made three wrong turns, each taking us to the Gandy Bridge, which we were not supposed to cross, forcing us to turn around each time. Then George found his bearings and directed Kenny toward Fourth Street where he watched for a sign.

"That's it." He pointed ahead to a one-story motel with the sign Grant Motel. We drove into a parking space beside the seedy L-shaped motel. Even in the dark, we could see that the building was in dire need of a coat or more of paint to restore it to its original white. Brown shutters and ledges framed the windows; a plastic chair in front of each door was the same dark color. Kenny went inside the office to pick up a key and then directed George to drive the car around behind the front building. Key in hand, Kenny walked through the complex and had the door unlocked by the time we parked in our designated space. He met George at the trunk, and they quickly gathered our luggage and took it inside.

By the time Sybil and I made our way into the dreary room, George and Kenny were exiting the closet where they had hung and deposited our bags.

"It's freezing in here," George said.

Kenny turned to look into the closet. "There's a heater back here," he said, and stepped back, bringing a dusty gray heater into the room. Talking in low voices, he and George stooped to examine the ancient piece of tin to see how to turn it on.

Kenny had turned on a dim overhead light, but it did little to brighten the gloomy room. Sybil sat down beside a brown table that held a small faded artificial flower arrangement and a lamp with a dingy shade. I turned the lamp on, but it was no help in illuminating the room's smoke-darkened walls. A brown and

41

rust colored spread covered a faux walnut finish bed. It really did not matter that much to Sybil and me, because our focus was on the reason for being here: the cure. We totally believed that this journey was one that would save her life. Any other time, we would have been uneasy in this seedy motel. But at this moment we were simply happy to be anywhere in the vicinity of hope, regardless of the dark conditions. There had definitely been no hope in the scrupulously clean and sterile oncology hospital.

We watched the pilots silently while they muttered suggestions to each other on how to operate the heating contraption. They were speaking too softly for us to hear. Evidently, the heater was not the only matter that disturbed them. One of them whispered, "I don't want to set these ladies in this motel. I'm not really happy with this place." It looked rough and shady to them. "We ought to have them put a chair in front of the door." It took several minutes to get the heater working. They reluctantly stood up to leave us.

We could not properly thank them for the extraordinary favor of their time and flying costs. Their willing spirit of generosity humbled me. Meekly I offered, "Could we take you out for a drink?"

After a quick glance at George, Kenny replied, "No, thanks. We have to fly."

I was embarrassed that I did not think about flying restrictions and wished that I had offered to buy their dinner instead. I was impressed by their professional efficiency and extremely grateful for their thoughtfulness. Sybil and I had to settle for giving them sincere thank-you hugs before they left us. It was sad to see the door close behind them.

"I have to go check us in at the desk," I said.

"I'm hungry," Sybil announced.

"Me, too."

"Ask someone up front if there is any place to eat nearby."

"I hope there is something within walking distance."

At the office, I had to press a buzzer before the clerk remotely unlocked the door and let me enter. This was not a good sign. The smiling white-haired woman, whom I later came to know as Mary, seemed quite at ease behind the counter. However, when she asked me to sign for a telephone and the TV remote control, I realized we should be cautious about our surroundings. Mary informed me that there was a coin laundry room for the guests to use. In addition to the soft drink machines, there was a machine there that sold powder. I was glad to hear that. We had packed lightly and would need to launder our clothes frequently.

I discovered that the motel owned some cottages behind the main building; these were rented to "snowbirds" escaping the extreme cold in the northern states. The motel's amenities were for their use as well as the roomers.

Mary said that she did not know of any restaurants nearby. Yet the next morning, I saw a Burger King next door, a family restaurant across the street, and another diner three doors down on the same block. Mary parked right beside the door that kept her locked inside her cubbyhole at night and probably never paid any attention to her outside surroundings. She suggested we call for pizza delivery.

"That sounds good. My daughter will like that."

I walked back into our room and held out the phone in my right hand. "Here's our telephone." And then I held out my left hand. "And here's our remote for the TV." We laughed.

I plugged the telephone in, and we laughed again when I realized that the cord fit so loosely in the wall outlet that in order to make a call, we needed to hold the cord firmly in the fixture to get a dial tone and then continue holding it there until the call was finished.

While we waited for the pizza, I poured wine into our plastic cups for a toast. "To your rehabilitation and good health!"

"I'll drink to that!" Sybil raised her glass and her voice. "I can't wait to get started on the treatments," she said with excitement. "I am so ready!"

We were happy and tremendously relieved to be in this place of promise. Neither of us had trouble sleeping that night.

It was not yet daylight when the telephone rang to wake us from our deep sleep. When I reached for it, the cord loosened from the outlet, and I had to jump up and push it back in to restore the power.

"Mom?" Randy's voice greeted me cheerfully.

"Randy, where are you?"

"I'm just across the bridge from St. Petersburg."

"Wow! You drove all night?" We did not expect him so soon.

"Yeah, but I stopped here for a nap a couple of hours ago."

"You must be exhausted."

"No, I'm okay," he assured me. "I'll come on over and bring you some coffee."

"Randy's here already?" Sybil asked in amazement.

"He's bringing coffee."

"I'm ready for that."

"Me, too." I was so relieved and proud that Randy came to be with us. "We had better get dressed before he gets here."

I dressed quickly, brushed my teeth, and cleansed my face before helping Sybil out of bed and into the bathroom. She sat next to the sink while I gave her a hand getting into her sweat suit. She partially dressed herself, and then I lifted her lame arm into the right sleeve. We made sure she had her anti-smoking patch. She was doing very well without cigarettes and had not even mentioned craving one. I put Sybil's washcloth, toothbrush, and toothpaste on the sink within reach of her good hand. Then I set out her makeup paraphernalia on nearby stool.

By the time Randy knocked at the door, we were fully dressed and ready for the day. Randy stood in the doorway with coffee cups in hand and a big smile on his face.

Sybil and I sipped our coffee gratefully. Hers was decaffeinated, however, because Randy was starting her on a new diet regimen.

"I'll call Joe's office for directions." Randy was looking at the telephone by the bed. When he reached for it, the plug came out of the wall. "What the ——?" he said, laughing.

"You have to hold the cord in and stand really still to get a connection."

Nancy gave Randy directions to 8085 Thirty-eighth Avenue North. "It's just over the bridge after a stoplight at Albertson's Grocery. Turn at the big red-hot sign onto a street between two buildings. This building is directly behind the building with the big red-hot." He had to ask about the "big red-hot" a couple times before he realized she was saying "big red heart."

Randy was equipped. He filled bottles with distilled water for him and Sybil. He had learned from Pat that the treatments caused dry mouth. Each of us took a book. I checked the tape recorder and made sure that it held a blank tape, and then I put it in the back seat for Sybil so that she could begin recording her experience.

In the daylight, we saw the family cafe across the four-lane street in front of the motel and opted for breakfast there.

A pleasant dark-haired server greeted us with a smile and then ushered us through the middle of the dining room to a booth that sat on a raised platform. I took Sybil's arm to help her maneuver a step upward and realized that this simple obstacle might be only one of many future hindrances she would have to face in the real world.

That first difficult step for her was a turning point for me. I learned to calculate distances and obstacles in advance so that I could help her. Unfortunately, there would be some instances in which I would miscalculate. Such times would be disconcerting for both of us. While we sat in the booth, Randy began to coach us about foods that helped fight cancer and build immune systems. Sybil had ordered oatmeal, a good choice according to his plan. The three of us decided to meet the diet challenge together.

The directions that Nancy gave Randy sounded simple, and they actually were, but the distance was much further than we anticipated. The scenery along the way was not very exciting. The small ranch homes bordering the streets seemed to have been built from one plan, distinguishable from one another only by varying shades of paint and slight modifications in landscaping. We were anxious to get Sybil started with the treatment and could not get there fast enough. I believed that every passing hour was important toward advancing her recovery.

Finally, we recognized the big red heart on a huge white banner covering the roof of a small building on the right side of the road. It was a good marker for the blind driveway between the two buildings. We turned into the drive and headed toward a simple but neat one-story structure behind the buildings. Randy drove directly toward the handicapped ramp in front of the clinic. Sybil and I got out and waited as he parked the car and came to help me lead her into the building. The large window that surrounded the glass entrance door presented a clear and open greeting. I let Randy hold Sybil's hand while I pulled the door open for them.

No one was standing duty behind the tall curved front desk when we walked into the Victorian-style lobby. Nancy was apparently in another part of the building. A deep plush burgundy sofa, loveseat, and chair offered seating in the room, though I soon found that it was less comfortable than it appeared. An antique sideboard held a silver coffee urn on one side of the room; beside it was a water cooler. The fresh cleanliness impressed me as we walked past the receptionist's station in search of assistance. We saw a gym filled with exercise equipment behind two glass doors to our left. I knew that Randy was making a mental note of the equipment and would find a way to use it. He always exercised, even if running was his only option.

We heard muffled voices and followed the sound down a quiet hall past empty offices, where other antique cabinets and shelves held unique glass and crystal collections from around the world. We later learned that Joe had traveled extensively during his long military career. At the end of the hall was a doctor's scale, and after a sharp left turn we found the large room from which the voices originated.

Over twenty recliners of varying dark colors lined two walls, and another dozen sat back to back in the center of the room.

Patients exchanging small talk occupied a few of the chairs. There was a broad white working space where two staff members were working busily. A short bald man with wire spectacles dressed in a white jacket acknowledged our presence with a nod. He continued working with a young, brown-haired nurse; he was concentrating on the task of carefully filling IV bottles.

Randy ushered Sybil to an end recliner and sat down beside her. Her eyes were bright with excitement. I realized the recliners were there only for the patients, so I remained standing. Moreover, the recliners were filling up swiftly. People of all ages and sizes filed into the room one at a time to fill the empty seats. We were fascinated with the activities revolving around us. The individuals represented all lifestyles. But I noticed that one thing they had in common was their obvious admiration of Joe DiStefano. It was easy to see that their belief in him and his treatment was genuine. None of their faces showed any sign of self-pity. Most of the patients were cheerful and friendly, and many clearly knew each other.

A white-haired lady rose from a navy blue recliner across the room, stopped at a baker's rack on the side wall, and picked up a couple of blankets and pillows before approaching us. She handed the spreads to my youngsters and placed a pillow on the arm of each chair

"I'm bringing you blankets today," she said pleasantly, "but after today, you're on your own." She smiled broadly and laughed.

Pat had forewarned us about chills following the treatments. The process raises the body's internal temperature to boost the immune system and stop cancer growth, but it causes the patient to feel chilled on the outside. Everyone had a blanket and a pillow to cradle the arm that would hold the IV.

"Thank you," we said in unison and smiled at the woman and at each other. The friendly icebreaker made us feel welcome. The room's pleasant atmosphere presented a stark contrast to the cold white corridors of the Spartanburg oncology clinic. I was so thankful that Sybil was in this friendly, warm space.

We watched Dr. Joe and the nurse, whom a patient called Jean, finish filling bottles and then start preparing patients for their infusions. A brass chain hung from the ceiling beside each chair, with a hook at the end to hold the bottle of serum and the tubes connected to the arm of the ailing patient.

There were patients with a variety of malignant tumors, but others suffered from heart disease. Those with heart problems came to the clinic for chelation therapy, which improves metabolic and circulatory function by removing toxic metals (such as lead and cadmium) and abnormally located nutritional metallic ions (such as iron) from the body. This is accomplished by administering EDTA, an amino acid.

DiStefano began administering chelation therapy for heart ailments many years before he began dispensing experimental aloe therapy for cancer patients. His orderly sterile clinic was a credit to the chelation profession.

After he and Jean had dispensed serum to all the patients, Joe came over to meet us. He knew who we were because he had expected us to be there on that morning. Randy stood and greeted him with a handshake. "I'm Randy Sechriest." He turned to introduce Sybil and me.

"We'll go down to the office to talk," he said. We followed him down the hall, but when he looked into his office, his wife, Georgiana, was at his desk, so he continued to the lobby.

Nancy had returned to the front desk. The caregiver with whom she had been chatting stood aside but watched and listened curiously while Joe consulted with us. As we would learn in the coming days, the man's father was one of the patients receiving Albarin.

"We got involved with Albarin through Dr. Ivan Danhof," Joe began. "Dr. Danhof had researched an extract of the aloe vera plant for some thirty odd years. He actually worked for a company that developed it for the treatment of feline leukemia. And after he made some discoveries about the extremely complex molecule and decided to put it into practice, he was looking for a clinic to run trials. And that's when I met him. He asked if we would like to participate, and we consented after visiting his research facility and his office at the University of Texas. The university actually had given him the original grant to study aloe vera, so we decided that we would go ahead and get people involved. We hope to publish some studies and ultimately get FDA approval.

"We have treated many patients, most of who are at stage four, with about two to six months to live. We have seen tumors shrink, prostates shrink, and so on. We have seen remarkable things. It doesn't work the same for everybody. But a majority of people have seen their cancer shrink and have more energy."

Joe's goal was to cure patients. He finished his consultation and took us to meet Dr. Daniel Mayer, a kind, silver-haired man with a receding hairline and a friendly twinkle in his eyes when he smiles broadly. Dr. Mayer is a physician and surgeon and also a former minister. He came out of retirement to work with Joe. He felt that Joe was doing such good work and believed it was a great thing to help with. Since Joe is not himself a medical doctor (though patients affectionately call him "Dr. Joe"), he needed someone with Dr. Mayer's qualifications to address physical conditions and prescribe medications.

At this time, Dr. Mayer told Sybil to stay on the medications she brought with her from Spartanburg: 2 mg of dexamethasone for swelling and Xanax as needed for anxiety. Later he would prescribe Percocet for her pain.

Joe did not make appointments. He took patients as they came. Without any mention of his fee, he led Sybil and Randy back to the recliners so they could begin treatment immediately. Joe worked from morning until night, never stopping to leave the building, not even for food. His priority was caring for his patients. Occasionally, some thoughtful patients or caregivers would bring him something to eat.

The following day, Georgiana asked me to write a check for $1,125 for the treatments. Joe's mind was on hope and healing, not money. The compassionate doctor was on a mission and sometimes gave care free of charge if a patient did not have enough money. Sybil, for example, was never billed for anything other than the original fee of $1,125.

I followed the three back to the treatment room. The doctor prepared formula for them while Sybil and Randy checked their blood pressure and weight. When they returned to their original seats, they surveyed the room and grinned at each other, happy to be participating with the other clients in Joe's trial. I waited until Joe came to begin the flow of fluid into their veins, and then I went back to the lobby to wait with other family members.

An hour later, I went to the treatment room to find my young ones wrapped tightly in their blankets. Sybil was sleeping peacefully in her blanket cocoon. Randy just looked up at me sleepily and grinned. The sight of them was bittersweet. I wanted to tuck them in with a goodnight kiss and find Sybil as healthy as she was when I did have them at home with me to tuck into bed at night. I was so relieved that the healing treatment was at last underway.

Dr. Joe chatted with patients as he worked. He gave them advice about their diet, offered information about supplements, and answered their numerous questions. The atmosphere was pleasant. Each person, with the exception of Randy, was afflicted with a life-threatening illness. Their common plight gave them a head start toward becoming acquainted.

When Sybil awoke, Randy came out to the lobby to get me.

"Sybil needs to go to the bathroom," he told me. "I'll wait here."

She smiled as I approached her. "How do you feel now?" I asked as I picked up her blanket to fold.

"Shaky and cold," she replied trembling, "and hungry."

I put the blanket and pillow back on the shelf and returned to help her rise from the recliner. Then I took her arm and led her slowly to the women's restroom and into the handicapped stall. She took hold of the rail, maneuvering on her own. I closed the door for her. "Let me know if you need help. I'll be right here." I sat on a narrow wooden bench nearby and waited.

As we left the building, Randy discovered that the best way to lead Sybil was to stand in front of her and take each of her hands in his. Each time he took one step back, she moved her facing foot forward, then he moved his other foot back and she moved hers forward. It was as if they were learning dance steps. It was touching to see my two children move together this way. We both walked with her this way from then on.

When I opened the back car door for her, she sat down trembling. "I've got to eat something."

"What can she eat?" I turned and asked Randy.

"We can stop at a Subway," he replied. "I saw one on the way over this morning."

Sybil, who missed hearing our exchange, called out from the back, "I need some food right now!" Her voice was panic stricken. It was the first sign of her urgency to eat immediately when hunger struck.

Randy and I exchanged serious glances. I turned toward the back seat so she could hear me explain. "Randy is going to stop at a Subway," I told her. "Will that be all right?"

She nodded. "That sounds good. I like sub sandwiches," she said gratefully. "but please hurry."

"It will take only a few minutes to get the sandwich. The shop is on our way home," I assured her. It occurred to me that part of her trembling panic might be nicotine withdrawal, so I promised to change her nicotine patch as soon as we got back to the motel.

Sybil waited anxiously while Randy and I went into the shop for our sandwiches. As soon as we were back in the car, Sybil grabbed her chicken sandwich on whole wheat and wolfed it down. Her trembling soon stopped. We decided that in the future we would prepare snacks for her so that she could keep some food in her system at all times. Thereafter we supplied her with plenty of fruits and nuts for sustenance between meals. It made a tremendous difference in her well-being during and after the Albarin treatments.

Sybil toyed briefly with the tape recorder, awkwardly holding it in her left hand and then slapping it down on the back seat with disdain. "My voice is gone," she announced somberly. She would never try again.

"Maybe you can make some notes on your laptop," I suggested. She did not respond. We both knew that she could only work with one hand, having watched as she typed short e-mail messages to friends and family.

Back at the shabby motel, which looked pitiful in broad daylight, Sybil went directly to bed. "I'm still sleepy," she announced. She lay on top of the covers fully clothed and was asleep in an instant.

"I'm going to go back to Joe's gym," Randy told me.

"Are you sure it will be okay?" I asked him. "Don't you think you should rest after the treatment?"

"I feel great, not the least bit sleepy," he assured me. "I'll call when I finish working out to talk about dinner. I can pick up something on my way back."

Suddenly alone, I decided it would be a perfect time to take advantage of the swimming pool. I had been anticipating the luxury (it was the only notable extravagance Grant's Motel had) since driving by it on our arrival the night before.

I chose a book from the small supply that Sybil and I had brought along and hastily slipped into a swimsuit that I probably would not need. Then I stepped quietly outside.

Surprisingly, the pool was clean and well kept. I sat in a chair at the umbrella table nearest the gate and opened the book. For a time, I stared at the first page without focusing. I could not concentrate for fear that Sybil would awaken and need me.

I walked briskly back to the room to find her sleeping peacefully in the same position as I had left her. The sight of seeing her resting peacefully reminded me of my innocent little girl of years past. Tears welled in my eyes, and I wanted to keep her within earshot, should she waken and need me. I ran back to poolside, which was no longer inviting, and swiped a lounge chair to bring back to the room so that I could sit comfortably near her. Her present condition rendered her as helpless as a small child, dependent on her mother for care and protection.

The narrow walk in front of our small room was not wide enough to accommodate the long reclining chair. This motel room, however, had a back door. (One could quickly escape unnoticed, if need be.) The ground was wet along the edge of the building, so I backed away from the building and settled comfortably between two shrubs, with a perfect view of Sybil on the bed.

I was barely past the first page of my book when my mobile phone rang, jerking me to attention. Quickly I hit the on button, looking to see that the noise had not awakened Sybil before I answered.

"Where are you?" A loud curious voice demanded.

I did not recognize the voice. "I'm in St. Petersburg, Florida," I replied, perplexed "Who ..."

Before I could finish my question, the caller blurted out, "Why the hell did he give me this number?" Then the phone went dead. Only months did I discover that the call was from Eddy, of Ron and Eddy's Restaurant. He thought he was calling my home and did not know that Sybil had left the Spartanburg hospital. He wanted to send her some homemade lemonade, which she loved, and had called to ask me to stop by to pick it up for her. He was just one of many in our community who wanted to do something nice for Sybil.

The cook's call was just the beginning of an onslaught of phone calls. Mike and Bill were giving out my number. It was not a cost-effective idea at a time, since both incoming and outgoing calls were billed to my telephone number.

I heard a moaning sound and rushed inside to see Sybil stretching her limbs like a kitten from a nap.

"Hi, Sleeping Beauty, how do you feel?" I asked expectantly.

"Good," she murmured contentedly, "but I want a bath and shampoo."

Relieved by her calm attitude, I went into the bathroom to run her a warm bath. As I did so, she disrobed on her own. After slipping her easily into the soapy water, I gathered clean clothes and cosmetics.

"Feels great." Sybil smiled pleasantly and settled to soak cheerfully until the water cooled. I sat nearby and waited.

"Guess it's time to get out," she told me, "the water is cold."

"Good sign." I reached for a large bath towel that I had placed nearby on the floor. Sybil held her slippery left arm toward me as I knelt on the floor against the tub to help her rise up. When I pulled on her arm, her body slid deeper into the tub. She could not help push herself up with the paralyzed side. Her body twisted and she cried out.

"Oh, I'm so sorry." Then I tried to lift her by reaching under her shoulders.

"No, no!" she screamed.

She was dead weight, and her naked wet body was too slick to hold onto. My second attempt was even more excruciating for her, as it put pressure on both her good and bad sides. She slid backward in the soapy slick tub.

"Oh, my gosh!" I was afraid I would hurt her. "I just don't know how to do this." I stopped and leaned back to survey the situation. "Wait a minute. Let me think." There were tears in her eyes, and I, too, wanted to cry. She was only inches from the edge. I thought this should be doable.

I put a large beach towel on the edge of the tub and knelt forward again. "If you can turn just enough so that the towel will slide under you, maybe I can raise you over the edge with the help of the towel." (*Like a piece of heavy furniture*, I thought.) "We are going to get you out of there." She looked up at me apprehensively. I was uncertain myself, but I had to try.

We managed to get the towel under Sybil's body. I don't know how we did it, strength from fear, I suppose, but I pulled the towel with one arm and turned the side of Sybil's body at the same time. She screamed and rolled up over the edge of the tub on top of me. I fell backward with her rolling out and down with me.

She was crying. I held her. "I am so sorry, baby; we won't do this anymore. No more bathtubs," I declared emphatically. "From now on you can do a sponge bath at the sink, and I'll help you wash your hair there, too." I realized I was shaking and took a deep breath. "What a scary lesson." I managed to push her off me and into a sitting position against the tub. I was then able to raise her up and gently lead her toward a nearby chair. There, with the aid of Sybil's good side, we set her upright again to put her clothes on.

Surprisingly, even after that ordeal, she was able to tie her shoes. That was a thrill. She had not been able to do that for a while. She sat upright and laughed.

"I think this ridiculous and scary episode deserves a drink." My watch displayed four-thirty. "It's five o'clock somewhere."

I poured us a glass of red wine. We made a toast to Joe's Albarin treatments, new bathing techniques, and Sybil's health. We recovered from the bathing ordeal and fell into a fit of laughter. We were still joking about the ridiculous bathtub scene when Randy called about dinner.

"Joe told me about Siam Garden, a Thai restaurant. His wife is very health conscious and particular about where she eats, and this is one of her favorites. She considers it one of the neatest and cleanest in the area."

"Just a minute, I'll ask Sybil." I looked at her. "What about Thai?"

"I don't know much about Thai food, but I'm starving. Randy will have to choose for me. Tell him to make it good."

"Did you hear her?" I asked.

"Yeah, I'll pick something. What about you?"

"Pick something for me, too. Spicy is good," I said.

The food was outstanding. For Sybil, Randy chose *bai ka pao* (chicken stir-fried with Thai basil, garlic, onion, and fresh mushrooms).

Randy and Sybil talked excitedly about their day at the clinic. Randy's enthusiasm was infectious. Our exchange was upbeat, for we had high hopes of success and a healthy future for Sybil. The ringing of the lame wall telephone interrupted us. Randy gingerly picked up the handset.

"Sybil, it's Bill," he announced and handed her the phone. He and I resumed our discussion without listening to Sybil's exchange with her husband. Suddenly the receiver came flying toward us. Randy ducked, but the device grazed his head as it zoomed by, pulling the cord from its flimsy connection.

Laughing nervously, Randy said, "Well, you don't have to hit *me*."

"That is the meaning of 'flying off the handle,'" I observed as Randy picked up the phone, "or in other words, 'flying off the cradle.'"

Randy, still laughing, spoke into a dead connection. "Bill, I don't think Sybil wants to talk to you right now."

Sybil cursed Bill under her breath. They had had an angry clash about finances. "The cord is threadbare," I commented. "Might as well break the handset, too."

Nevertheless, she quickly let go of the hostility, and we were soon laughing again. It had been quite a day!

Later Sybil confided in me, without going into details, that she feared they might have to sell some of their property to pay Bill's taxes. I did not ask for nor did she volunteer the reason. Bill is self-employed, and business was always slow during the winter months. It was an added strain for her to bear during an already stressful time. Their conversation this evening was the straw that broke the camel's back. She had been relatively patient up to now about both her illness and the financial burden.

I knew first hand that she had only just recently reinstated her life and health insurance policies. At this time, having the health insurance was a blessing, for otherwise there would be medical as well as tax burdens.

Fortunately, the three of us were ready to adjust to whatever circumstances were to befall us. The small motel room where George and Kenny delivered Sybil and me was tight quarters, so when we added a cot for Randy to the mix, it became wall-to-wall sleeping space with very little walking space. The good news was that Sybil could often maneuver herself from the bed to the nearby bathroom on her own, depending on the position her body was in when she awoke.

Unfortunately, Randy snores loudly, but having the cot beside the bed made it easy for me to kick the cot and shake him. That usually provided short relief. Occasionally, when the kicking did not work, Sybil would call out to him, "Randy! Randy! Get up!"

"Wha—what?" He would rise up, sleepily curious, without hearing what she said. We would not answer, and he would lie back down to sleep silently for a while before beginning to snore again. He never remembered the incident the next day. She enjoyed the performance.

Every night at bedtime and upon waking during the night, I prayed, "Dear God, please clear, heal, and cure her." My faith in God had never been stronger, and I firmly believed that He would indeed cure her.

On the second day of treatment, Jean greeted Sybil with a handful of papers and a wide smile. "Guess what you got today." She held the messages out to Sybil. "Fax greetings from your fan club."

"Where are *my* letters?" Randy asked playfully.

"You didn't get any," Jean said. "But there is something else for Sybil." She pointed to a huge flower arrangement that sat in the corner nearby and plucked the card from for Sybil.

"And my flowers? Are you hiding them?" Randy teased.

"Didn't get any of those either. Guess you don't have a fan club," she retorted good-naturedly.

Thus began a daily ritual with the three of them. Fax notes, flowers, and cards continued to arrive at the clinic until we acquired another address. The cheerful banter between Randy and Jean lasted throughout his treatment program at the clinic.

Sybil told Jean about our stressful bathtub episode and asked whether she could use the bathroom shower at the clinic.

"Of course you can. Any time you want," she replied kindly. "And if there is anything else you need, all you have to do is ask."

Randy could not let that one go. "What about me, Jean. What are you going to do for me?"

"Randy, Randy," she chirped, "it's all about you." Then her voice changed to a warning tone. "Maybe I can come up with something for you."

"Never mind," he laughed, "you would probably use a dull needle for my injection."

"Thanks for the idea." She grinned as she walked away.

The following day I packed bath supplies and a change of clothes. After Sybil's treatment, I led her to the bathroom and into the shower stall. I helped her take her clothes off and then squeezed some shampoo into her good left hand. While she was shampooing, I put a soapy washcloth over the handicap rail within reach. She held herself steady by hooking her right arm onto the rail and bent her head downward. I adjusted the water temperature to spray her hair and then waited for her to work the shampoo through her short locks. After helping her with the rinse process, I handed her the soapy cloth.

"You're on your own now. Just let me know when you need me to dry you off and help you dress."

"Okay, Mom, go sit."

Seeing that she had good footing, I went to the bench and picked up the book that I had laid there.

Soon she declared happily, "I'm ready. I feel so much better."

I could have sworn she was walking better when we left the building that day. We took advantage of her high spirits to stop by a health food store to pick up supplies. We packed Sybil's protein and fruit in a flowered cosmetic bag. The small zippered bag also held a bottle of water and her meds. Each day we tucked the supplies in the left side of her recliner so she would have them at the ready when hunger hit, which usually happened quickly and vigorously. On a few rare occasions, we miscalculated the portions. Such slip-ups provoked anguishing panic attacks in Sybil and threw her into alarming tantrums. But aside from those fits of hunger anxiety and occasional upsets for other reasons, she was exceptionally cheerful.

It was a happy day for Sybil when her mother-in-law called unexpectedly one weekend. Neither Sybil nor I had given further thought to Lib's trip to Florida since her hospital visit in Spartanburg. We were therefore surprised that she was calling for directions to our motel. Her host friends were bringing her to visit.

We knew our living conditions were shabby, but our purpose was to be in St. Petersburg for healing not luxury. The seedy motel happened to be a necessary part of the program for the time being. But after Lib's request to drop in on us, I saw the dingy surroundings from a visitor's perspective. If seen as a reflection of the clinic, it might seem that we were dealing with quacks there. I hoped not.

Instead of talking about the embarrassing surroundings, I looked around the crowded interior space and suggested to Sybil and Randy that we take the table and chairs outside and visit there. Randy agreed and hoisted the table up to maneuver over the end of the bed and through the door. I moved a chair outside and then led Sybil to a seat at the table while we arranged a sitting area around the table in the parking lot.

Lib's hosts, a former minister and his wife, insisted on buying our lunch. While Randy and the minister drove to Boston Market for a fried chicken dinner with all the fixings, Lib and I hulled a basket of strawberries that she brought along from the Strawberry Festival.

It was a very pleasant luncheon break. Sybil was her cheerful self. She remained seated, and the only evident sign of her illness was a slight awkwardness in eating with her left hand. I think even that was probably only recognized by Randy and me.

I forgot about the gloomy room until it became necessary for me to escort Lib to the bathroom. *Oh, well! What the heck!* I thought to myself. *It is what it is.* So I led her into the dark room without saying a word. Those living conditions, after all, did nothing to change the plan of salvation.

During one of his telephone calls, Bill informed Sybil that Dr. Corso was leaving messages on Sybil's answering machine in North Carolina. "He wants you to call him, Sybil."

"I'm not going to call him. There is nothing more for us to discuss with Dr. Corso. I'm happy where I am now."

Our morning drives to the clinic were happy hours. Randy often tuned the radio to a popular music station and challenged us to name the vocalists as the music played:

"I write the songs that make the whole world sing ..."

"Barry Manilow," Randy declared.

"You are the sunshine of my life ..."

"Stevie Wonder," Sybil chimed.

"Baby, I'm-a want you, Baby, I'm-a want you, you're the only one I care enough to hurt about ..."

"I don't know. I have no idea."

Sybil tried to help me with a clue. "Mom, it's a carbohydrate."

"A carbohydrate? I have no idea."

Sybil and Randy laughed, and together said, "Bread."

"Bread?" I thought they were putting me on.

Finally, one morning, we heard "Strangers in the night, exchanging glances ..."

"Mom, you know this one," Randy declared.

"You are dating me, for sure," I answered. "Frank Sinatra."

It was fun to be playing with my kids again. The game made our ride fun.

Sybil and Randy easily made new friends in the treatment room at the clinic. Patients filled the therapy chairs, but there were never more than nine people in the lobby and often there were none. When I found myself alone in this strange setting of sickness, my mind inevitably rushed back to Sybil's healthier days and back to happier days that Sybil and her brothers shared with other friends.

Take Me Back

Let me do this again with a better ending

In their youth, Sybil and her brothers happily played baseball with their community playmates on weekends. Our front yard, a centrally located large open space, was the neighborhood baseball diamond. And our house was home to one third of the baseball team.

Sybil kept pace with both the boys and girls. Her natural curly hair frizzled during vigorous exercise. Since it was impossible to keep her hair smooth and untangled when she was so active, I suggested that we cut her hair short. She eagerly shared the plan with her paternal grandmother next door, who promptly voiced her disapproval. Sybil wanted to please everyone, so she tried to find a compromise.

"Mommy, you can cut my hair in the back," she innocently confided in me, "and then Granny can't see that it is cut."

However, I defied my mother-in-law's wishes and chose a cute pixie cut for her. I have a delightful photograph of that period that captures an impishly sweet child.

It was also about this time that Sybil made a startling discovery. "Mommy! Mommy!" She ran through the back door crying frantically, "My bowels are moving!" Both her hands were holding her heart where she felt a thumping movement.

"It's okay, honey," I put my hand over hers, "this is your heart. It will keep beating just like that all of your life."

When Sybil and her twin brother, Michael, went to their first day of school, I was very emotional. The teacher took them by the hand and drew them toward a circle with other small students. They were taking their first steps toward independence, learning things that would help them make their way through life without me. I would now have to develop a strong faith for the times when they were not in my sight. My little ones were already leaving the nest to soar into the vast wilderness of the unknown. My wings of protection could no longer spread wide enough to keep them from harm. I faced that same sadness when their younger brother Randy had his first day of school.

When tears started to sting my eyes, I would sneak away from the group of children to seek comfort from a dear father figure who owned a restaurant only a block away from the school. "Pop" always said the right thing, and I was able to dry my eyes and return with renewed optimism. My young ones did not miss me at all. Two of their classmates were next-door neighbors, and a few others were in their Sunday school class. They were thrilled to be in a circle with their friends.

Sybil made friends quickly and easily wherever she went. Her ready smile and curiosity offered a listening ear to stranger and friend alike. She established loyal friendships, many of them lifelong. Lynn, the youngster next door, became one such friend.

Using their lively imaginations, Sybil and Lynn created their own private *Bonanza* in the wooded area that separated their houses. Adam and Little Joe were their idols. They would spend hours on their "ranch," a huge tree stump that sat safely within my sight and hearing distance. Lynn went on later to build her real *Bonanza* horse ranch in Colorado but that did not interrupt her ongoing friendship and regular communication with Sybil.

Sybil had her girlfriends and boys that were good friends, but she always confided her innermost secrets to her most trusted and loyal companions, her loving pets. She loved animals and was never without a dog to talk to. She whispered her intimate thoughts to Blackie, Dober, Tinker, Candy, and Zach as they joined the family, one after another.

Home was ideal for the family. Just as the twins had the first birthday of their teens my husband was transferred to Forest City. It is a small town nestled in the foothills of the western North Carolina Mountains, 120 miles west of our Lexington home. The youngsters were not happy about moving away from their friends and the place they knew as home.

Fortunately, Sybil and her two brothers met a new group of friends right away. "Kick the can" was the game for that summer season in the new neighborhood. Their new friends introduced them to the recreation center, which had a swimming pool and gymnasium. There was a drugstore, a movie theatre, and a church in town, all within a mile. Now they were "uptown" and had an entire summer to become acquainted with their surroundings.

When the Cool Springs Middle School opened in the fall, they already knew many of their classmates from their summer initiation in the community. They and their classmates paraded cheerfully down the street after school to the popular drugstore soda fountain only a few blocks away. They crammed into the booths at Smith's Drugs, where they laughed and giggled between bites of their favorite snack, "oak cake shake base" (an oatmeal cookie smothered with milk shake flavored ice cream). Even after they moved on to East High School, the siblings and their friends enjoyed the same after-school pleasure on days that they did not have cheerleading, basketball, or football practice.

Sybil bonded with a group of happy girls that shared her interests, such as ... boys, of course. Huddled in the hall with the "in" group of new friends, they giggled about boys. Sybil listened to them discuss whom she should have for a boyfriend. Of course, they had already claimed their own choices from the previous year, so those boys were off limits.

A short, sandy-haired fellow strutted proudly toward them,

head thrown back confidently. One of the girls nodded toward him, "How about Pat Jobe?" she suggested.

Sybil looked in the direction of her gesture, "Him?" she asked incredulously when she saw the young man. "No way!"

Unfortunately, he read her lips, and his proud expression collapsed. Neither of them would ever forget that incident.

It came as no surprise that Sybil tried out for the cheerleader squad and made the team. My employer at the time, however, was upset. "Your daughter made cheerleader and my daughter did not," he complained. That was when I realized that her new school was much larger than her former county school. Competition would be greater here. She proved up to the challenge and passionate about the cheerleading, which she continued throughout middle school and high school.

Mike, Randy, and a group of their classmates were members of an after school basketball league, the BYBA, (Backyard Basketball Association.) It was organized by sports nut, Tommy Hicks because he could still play then. All the members had basketball goals in their yards. They took turns on the home courts. Sybil and her co-cheerleaders followed the BYBA from house to house to cheer for them.

Perky young Sybil was pretty and popular. She was a storybook teenager: chosen for the homecoming court, the key club calendar, yearbook staff, and senior class secretary. I have flashes of Sybil rushing in and out during those exciting and hectic teen years, including a bittersweet memory of her first date with a young man whose mother drove them to a "coffeehouse" dance at the First Methodist Church, chaperoned by a group of parents.

Our family furniture business was only a mile from the middle of town beside the "Welcome to Forest City" sign.

Sybil's first part-time job was at the Cracker Barrel restaurant. She truly had fun as a server and always had quick comebacks when the regulars teased her. One such customer, a successful realtor, teased her daily and always left a quarter tip, no matter the size of his tab. When he passed away years later, she dropped a quarter in his coffin at the funeral parlor.

The shopping malls and Wal-Mart had not yet invaded the safety of the downtown community. A hardware store, clothing stores, gift shops, pharmacies, newsstands, grocers, a movie theatre, churches, and department stores lined the Main Street strip. The community atmosphere fostered and nourished young relationships that would remain steadfast into and throughout adulthood.

Sybil was excited when she was accepted at Lenoir Rhyne College in nearby Hickory. Following her high school graduation, she spent the summer working at Cracker Barrel and planning for college.

She took her loving community spirit to Hickory and easily expanded her ever-growing circle of treasured and loyal friends.

She warmed instantly to her first roommate, Marce Snyder, a northerner from Ohio. They had fun with the "north and south" during their lifelong friendship. I felt that their bonding played a major part in Sybil's acclimation to living away from home.

Her father and I were delighted by a letter she wrote to us soon after she settled in at Lenoir Rhyne: "I am very happy here. Haven't any regrets whatsoever. It really is a great place. I am really looking forward to my next four years. It scares me to think that I almost gave it all up. This is also a letter to thank you for everything. It is also to say I am sorry for past disappointments. I hope there are no more in the future. I hope that I only give you pride and happiness in the future." (She did just that.) "Thank you for helping me through difficult times and giving me years of happiness. I know I have the greatest parents in the world and no one else can come close. Thanks for everything to both of you. Your favorite daughter, Sybil."

Her teenage waitress experience in Forest City served her well during college. Del Rozelle hired her to help him open McGuire's Pub, a new bar and grill in Hickory. It is a dimly lit eatery below street level on a downtown corner. The interior features lots of dark polished wood and an array of memorabilia. The opportunity was a challenge that she met skillfully. Sybil helped create the friendly relaxed atmosphere that still exists in the eatery. Sybil brought in college friends to work with her, including Jayne, who worked as host, server, and bartender there.

When they finished college, Randy and Sybil joined our family furniture business as managers of a branch store in Iron Station, North Carolina. They managed the business well, in spite of an occasional brother-sister squabble. Randy was technically the boss, and while Sybil yielded to courteous supervision, she did not tolerate scolding from her brother.

While living and working in Iron Station, Sybil fell in love with and married Bill Yount, a close friend of Randy's. Later, when we closed the Iron Station store, Sybil, Randy, and Bill joined us in our Forest City location. The young married couple soon began their family.

Their sons, Brian and David, started playing baseball on a T-ball team and continued through Little League and high school. David even went through college on a baseball scholarship. Sybil was their loudest cheerleader in the stands at every game. I was with her at some of them.

She and I were leaving the stands at one of those games when I saw that her gait was not quite normal. It was not exactly a limp; it was more like a weight-shifting shuffle. She seemed to favor her right leg, swaying slightly as she leaned more heavily on her left. It looked unnaturally awkward.

"Sybil, what is wrong with your legs?"

"My leg just gives way now and then," she replied offhandedly.

"I didn't notice this problem during our trip." We had recently spent a wonderful week together at Pompano Beach, Florida, and a three-day cruise to Nassau. It was a fun holiday, with lots of laughter. We had been relaxed and happy.

"Oh, it just comes and goes," she replied casually.

"Well, if it keeps happening, you'd better see a doctor."

"I have an appointment with Dr. Gill coming up. I'll ask him about it," she said.

Later she reported, "He told me to do some exercises."

A few weeks later, I noticed that the problem persisted. "Are you doing the exercises?" I asked.

She shrugged and nodded slightly but moved to another subject. She was young and healthy, so, like her, I surmised that the doctor knew what was going on. But I wondered why she was still favoring her right leg, especially when climbing steps or walking up an embankment.

That November, our family began getting ready for the holiday season. Each year Sybil seemed to add new projects to her annual traditions. She made pound cakes for Bill's customers (a list that kept growing), candy for her friends and family (a list that kept growing), and served Thanksgiving dinner for family and others (more and more each year), not to mention participating in numerous Christmas parties and dinners.

Sybil and I were together as often as we could arrange it. We made frequent trips to Sam's Club in Spartanburg. On the November trip, we gathered supplies for all the holiday cooking and baking. She and I bought in bulk so we could share.

"I'll buy the cleaning supplies while you get the baking products you need for cakes and candy," I told her. "We won't get lost, I can find you by your cough."

She reminded me that the cough was simply due to allergies. "We're going to get a new filter installed at the house. It supposedly cleans the air of dust and pollen."

During the holidays, Sybil's kitchen turned into a caterer's domain, a bakery, and a candy factory.

Thanksgiving dinner always included Bill and Sybil's sons, mothers, other family members, and friends, including Jayne and Ward as well as Bud and Teresa Crotts. In addition, Sybil was especially conscious of anyone who may not have had anywhere to go for Thanksgiving dinner and opened her home to welcome them for that celebration dinner.

In addition to her popular potato casserole, Sybil always baked a ham and made gravy and dressing. Bill deep-fried a turkey, and Bud and Teresa Crotts brought a baked turkey along with Teresa's cranberry salad. Jayne and Ward brought appetizers and special gourmet sides. Ward carved the ham and turkey. I made my popular asparagus casserole.

Sybil was the center of everything, keeping a close watch on bread and dressing in the oven while greeting everyone cheerfully, hugging, joking, and laughing. She was a cheerful host, always thrilled when her house filled with guests.

The day after Thanksgiving, Sybil and Jayne started working on their annual tradition: making candy for a Christmas list of family and friends. The task kept them busy for the entire holiday weekend.

I stopped in during the day for a glass of wine and to watch the comedy. And comedy it was. Neither of the girls would bother to dress for the day. Sloppy sweats, no makeup, hair uncombed. They were barely up from bed before starting their assembly line for the day. Chocolate melting on the stove was used to cover cream-wrapped cherries, syrup-shrouded pecans, coconut rolls, and almonds. Sybil spread them out on the waxed paper; Jayne dripped the chocolate.

I never let myself be drawn into anything except the joking and laughter, though I did quietly volunteer to pick up supplies if they ran out of something.

Once the candy manufacturing was out of the way, Sybil began baking the pound cakes for Bill's customers.

Amid the hustle and bustle at the end of 2000, Sybil was ever mindful that her son Brian would soon become a father. In mid-December, I took her excited telephone call.

"I'm a grandmother! It's a girl!" This was one of the happiest thrills of Sybil's life. "Her name is Hannah Marie. Being a grandmother is going to be great! She looks like Brian. Do you want to go see her?"

"Of course I do! When can we go?"

"Today!" Though she had been up all night, she could hardly wait to see the baby again.

Only a week after their grandchild was born, Bill was sick with a virus for a few days. When he recovered, Sybil became ill. We assumed that she had the same virus as her husband.

When our family gathered for Christmas Eve, Sybil was still not feeling well, but she joined our small crowd anyway, looking pale and drawn. This celebration was not as joyous as usual. Sybil was quiet and out of character, and Randy was absent, having gone to his favorite fishing place at Spring Creek, Florida, with a new girlfriend.

I was sad when Sybil left early. She was my "winding down" partner. She usually stayed to finish the evening with me, helping clear away the clutter of paper and dirty dishes. Then we would sit for one more glass of wine before she went home to greet Santa for her sons. This year was different. The evening ended with a strange sense of foreboding.

Christmas Day included the big family, my mother, siblings, nieces and nephews, and our Christmas Eve group. Sybil usually rode with me to Lenoir, where Mother lived with my older brother and his wife. However, when I drove over to pick her up on Christmas morning, she was still wearing only sweats and no makeup.

"I feel better today than yesterday, and I really want to go, but I just don't feel like I can ride up there and back." Her eyes lacked their lovely sparkle, and her radiant smile was missing. "Bill wants to ride with you, though."

I was sorry to leave her alone on Christmas Day. "I'll be glad for Bill to go with me. He can drive. I'm sure he doesn't want me to." I looked at Bill, who was amusedly nodding in agreement.

No one expected Sybil's illness to last long. But within a month, we were sitting with extremely ill cancer patients, and Sybil was sharing their fate. *I cannot reverse this process*, I thought.

The Clinical Environment
A place of refuge and comradeship

Among the new friends that Sybil and Randy made in the treatment room at the clinic was Bob Becks, a fifty-eight-year-old roofer from Clearwater, Florida. Bob was a walking testimonial for Joe. He was one of the success cases that Pat had mentioned. It was encouraging to see the man enjoying the positive result of the treatment.

Bob had a softball-sized tumor in his neck. It was too late for surgery. Bob believed that chemicals and radiation *cause* cancer, so it did not make sense to him to have mainstream treatments. He started taking the Albarin treatment in December, about a month before Sybil. "It stopped the tumor right in its tracks," he was fond of telling new patients.

Sybil and Randy especially enjoyed teasing a hypochondriac whom I will call Fred. Fred tried every alternative cure he heard about and would do so whether or not he needed it. He had only minor ailments, not cancer, but he was scared. When he first found a seat next to Randy, he was undergoing chelation therapy. Then he became excited after Randy explained the positive effects of Albarin. The following day when Sybil and Randy arrived for treatment, Fred had switched from chelation to Albarin. "I can feel this going through my arms. Do you feel this going through your arms?" he asked them.

Sybil punched Randy and shook her head.

"No," Randy said, "We don't feel a thing."

Later, when Fred's bottle was almost empty, he asked, "Do you get a headachy feeling?"

Randy, who was sitting between Fred and Sybil, looked at her and winked. She grinned when he turned back to Fred. "No, Fred, we never get a headache. Don't feel a thing." They also fibbed to Fred about chills and did not explain their blankets to him.

Each day Fred was there, Sybil and Randy came to the car laughing about Fred's fear for the day.

"Poor Fred," I told them. "He probably hasn't slept a night since you met him."

"There's nothing seriously wrong with him," they told me. "And he always wants to sit with us." They looked forward to sitting beside him, anxious to see what the malady of the day would be. Fred gave them descriptions of the various alternative treatments he had tried for prevention.

My youngsters were eager to hear Joe's advice to other patients.

"Joe," asked one patient, "what do you think about the cayenne pepper cure?"

Joe stopped and answered patiently. "Good for you, good for the bloodstream. People who take enough cayenne probably don't have to think about Viagra."

We were all concerned about patients who were extremely ill, as was the case with a young man in his late teens. They called him "the kid." His case tugged at our heartstrings.

I was waiting in the lobby with two other caregivers when the kid arrived, accompanied by his father, mother, and girlfriend. He was bald from chemotherapy and trembled as he walked cautiously between his parents. The girlfriend trailed a few steps behind them. They spoke softly to Nancy, who led them down the hall to wait privately in Joe's office for their introduction. Some time later, the father came back alone and sat down on the empty love seat. A man seated in one of the wing chairs asked about the boy.

The distressed man replied, "The doctors said he wouldn't live and sent him home to die." The man's voice broke, and he could say no more. His eyes filled with tears. No one asked further questions. Later we learned that the cancer had spread throughout the young man's body. Joe came in on some days when the clinic was closed to give the young man additional treatments at no extra charge. The kid had to enter the hospital often for pain treatment. We heard that the girlfriend returned to Ohio, and shortly thereafter, the father suffered a nervous breakdown and returned home, leaving the mother to cope alone with her desperately ill son. A couple of weeks later, the mother and son were compelled to return to their hometown for the young man's last days. All the staff and patients mourned his passing.

The medical center offered flexible times for the patient treatments. That practice freed both the patients and their caregivers from the pressure of having to make scheduled appointments, as happens in traditional medical centers. Sybil usually chose to go to the clinic early in the morning, but occasionally it was more practical for her to go later in the day. It might seem that such an accommodating practice would create a "bottleneck" for patients, but that was not the case. It seemed to work out naturally that patients did not have to wait for a seat in the treatment room. There was room for caregivers in the lobby. The flexibility also allowed both the clients and their families to meet different people coming at varying hours.

During one early morning wait, I met Harold Harmon, a tall, pleasant Kentucky construction worker. Harold had a ruddy complexion, strong hands toughened from hard work, and a quick but brief smile. His father entered the clinic for prostate cancer treatment and was beginning to recover. He was frustrated with his sister-in-law, also a cancer patient in the clinic, for not only was she not eating healthfully but she also smoked steadily and relied more heavily on pain medication than the Albarin solution.

She often skipped days of treatment. He was caretaker for both of them, but he felt helpless when she ignored proper care. The three of them were rooming in a trailer park.

On one of our afternoon visits, we met Deedy Fincher. Deedy was a beautifully dressed middle-aged woman adorned with makeup and bright jewelry. She made a commanding grand entrance through the lobby, blonde head held high. She had a noticeable limp but carried a heavily laden grocery bag. She slowed as she walked by Nancy. "Where's Dr. Mayer? I've brought him some fruit, and I want to make sure he gets it." She was still talking as she entered the hall. "He never stops to eat." The receptionist did not have a chance to answer before Deedy disappeared down the hall. "Where's Dr. Mayer?" she asked loudly of no one in particular. On another occasion, she sailed through the lobby in the same cocky way, leading a furniture delivery man who was wheeling in a new recliner on a hand truck. She sent him back to the truck to bring in another for the clients.

Deedy's take-charge attitude annoyed me. She seemed haughty and arrogant. But I learned to appreciate her generosity and to discount the demanding way she displayed that bigheartedness. We became good friends. Her proud manner suggested, "Stand aside so that I can give you something that you need."

When she discovered Sybil in the treatment room, she thought that oxygen would be good for her. Before she sat down for her own Albarin infusion, she went to the wall where oxygen tanks were standing and rolled one over to Sybil and connected it for her. Deedy had been a nurse for a number of years, and it was evident that she had been a good one, in spite of her forceful style of nurturing.

There was an attractive gray-haired woman whose nature was opposite of Deedy. She sat quietly in the reception room waiting for her husband to complete his treatment. She always had a book and kept her head down, obviously wanting to be alone.

Sometimes, the extra time it took for Sybil to shower after her treatment delayed lunch. Randy and I had learned the hard way to make sure that she had enough food in her snack pack to last until the noon meal. Even so, timing was occasionally close, and we would go to a nearby health food store, which had an adjoining restaurant that provided prompt pick-up service and convenient seating for Sybil. The patrons and clerks there were thoughtful, and she felt comfortable.

By the time we returned to the motel after treatment, showering, and lunch, Sybil was always exhausted. She fell onto the bed right away, grabbing the remote control so that she could tune in to her regular soaps, *The Young and the Restless* and *As the World Turns*. Her Bible and current novel were always on a bedside table. She listened to the programs as she catnapped and read in between.

Mail, fax messages, and gifts continued to come regularly to the clinic. We bought note cards so that Sybil could send thank-you messages. It was a daily ritual that the two of us did together. Even though I physically wrote the messages for her, Sybil made sure the words were hers. If I suggested wording that she did not feel like saying, she would correct me.

I subscribed to the local Internet service, Ozline, and checked e-mail messages on Sybil's laptop computer while she rested. Every day, someone mentioned a new prayer list including her name. With so many prayers, I saw no way she could lose this horrendous battle.

Sybil and I met one of our neighbors in the motel, a middle-aged snowbird from Michigan who was staying in St. Petersburg through February. The morning after we met, she brought a bowl of hot oatmeal for Sybil. The nice surprise came with a discovery: there were mini-kitchens in some of the motel quarters. Wow! We needed one of those.

I went right away to the office and asked Mary, "Do you have a room with a kitchen available?"

"Not now," she said, "but if the couple across the parking lot from you leaves this weekend, you can move in there. They said they would be checking out on Saturday."

"Great! Put us down for it." We were planning to find a

different place for us to live, but until that happened, we could at least upgrade from a small room to a kitchen suite. The upgrade had the same drab furniture, and the kitchen was a tiny cubicle, but it would be an improvement nonetheless.

It was an exciting day at the clinic when Harold's father got the news that his cancer was in remission and possibly cured. He and Harold were to go home, and the brother of Harold's sister-in-law would take over as her caretaker.

When he left, Harold gave me a list of accommodations that he was looking into and would no longer need. While Sybil and Randy were in the treatment room, I studied the Harmon rental list, read the classified ads, made calls, and investigated properties. In addition, I ran other errands to pick up supplies.

One evening, we decided it was time to go out for dinner instead of bringing food to the room. We chose a seafood place, Crabby Bill's. The restaurant had a long zigzag handicap ramp with a railing leading up to the entrance. This was good for Sybil, who was able to walk by holding onto the rail instead of Randy or me. Once we were inside, however, there was a long dining hall almost full of patrons. Randy and I followed the head server between the crowded tables toward an empty space near the back of the restaurant. We took Sybil by the hand between us and walked slowly to the vacant table. Sybil's first comment after we helped her onto the bench seat at the long table was, "People are staring at me." Randy and I were upset to see her this way. I so wish I had had the foresight to suggest we leave before taking the long walk through this restaurant. Surely we could have found easier access for Sybil at another place.

She used her one good hand to toy with the flounder on her plate, having lost her appetite during this ordeal. Randy and I tried to cheer her up. Her infirmity bothered her more when it was seen through the eyes of strangers who dared to stare at her. We never knew where this might happen. The experience dampened all our spirits, but we tried to keep our dialogue light and ignore other diners. "We'll show them in a few weeks when you are able to walk in here alone with your head held high."

Randy had more difficulty staying still in the drab motel room than Sybil and I. The gym was a blessing for him, because he was accustomed to working out every day. Occasionally, he went to a movie in the afternoon. We had our books, and Sybil had her soaps to occupy her when she was not sleeping.

Richard Turk, a friend of Randy's, had a home nearby in Palm Harbor. Richard invited Randy to visit with him for a weekend break and hang out by the pool. Sybil and I drove him over to meet Richard.

I had come to depend on my son for reassurance. Without him, I felt uncertain and nervous about Sybil.

The telephone calls kept coming, mostly on my cell phone. Some friends had just discovered that she was desperately ill, others knew beforehand and wanted regular updates, and everyone wanted us to know how much they cared and that they were offering prayers for us. My phone bill was soaring, because I did not have a plan covering Florida. We gathered all the e-mail addresses that we could and switched from phone to Internet.

Sybil's first e-mail read: Dear friends and family, I am grateful for your thoughts, prayers, and messages. I cannot write or e-mail because of the numbness in my right side, but I can tell my Mom what to do. I feel like I am where I should be, led through the power of prayer and thoughts from friends, family, and community. All this is taking me into each new day with renewed spirit and determination to make each day better. SYB."

Using e-mail reduced our telephone calls by half. We continued to send out weekly updates.

Mary told us that we could move across the parking lot to the larger room with a mini-kitchen. The sink, range, table, and chairs were crowded into the tiny space, leaving only a narrow aisle to get to the bed in the adjoining room.

On our first evening in the new space, Sybil started to get up from a chair and suddenly fell between the chair and the bed. My heart leapt as I jumped up in fright.

She saw my expression of fear and reassured me, "I'm okay … I'm okay!"

Once again, we faced with the challenge of lifting her up. Helping her up was again difficult, but not nearly as hard as the bathtub incident. The cramped space she fell into made it simpler. She used her good left side to hold onto the chair that was now against a wall, and I used the bed as a brace to keep from sliding backward as I pulled the dead weight of Sybil's bad side. The episode shook both of us, but we laughed with relief that she was not injured.

The tiny kitchen had space for Randy's blender at the sink. He treated us to his healthy "green drink" for breakfast.

I had doubts when I saw the green drink. Fortunately, it had a much better taste than I expected. I actually enjoyed it.

The Green Drink

> 6 oz. apple juice
> 2 oz. aloe vera juice
> Yogurt
> Almonds
> Bananas and or other fruit
> Honey
> Powdered greens (chlorophyll)
> (And other, if desired—use your imagination)

Sybil was now having trouble getting up during the night to go to the bathroom. It bothered her when she needed my help. Sometimes she could manage alone because the bed was close to the wall and she could swing over the side.

"I don't mind getting up when you need me," I told her.

"But I don't want you to have to. If I don't get turned around the wrong way in the bed, there's no problem."

"A walker could help you maneuver better on your own when you have that dilemma," I suggested cautiously.

"No," she said firmly. I said no more about it at that time. But a day or two later, as I led her from her treatment by stepping backward with her forward steps, I mentioned the subject again. "Sybil, I am sure you could manage by yourself if you had a walker. A walker would simply be taking my place, because I only keep you steady as you walk."

She looked at me, thinking about what I said, possibly imagining the process. Then she sighed and reluctantly agreed. "Okay, I'll try to use one."

She held to the top of the car door to swing herself inside. Then she sat, with her right numb arm swinging loose in the door opening, not realizing that it was still outside the car. I waited until she looked down at it. "Oh," she said, grinning at me and laughing as she picked her numb arm up with her left hand. This happened quite often, and I would always wait for her to bring her arm inside rather than pick it up for her. I had the feeling that if I moved her arm for her she would no longer see it as amusing.

Sybil settled back into her seat, and I fastened the seat belt she pulled up from her left side. "I'll go back inside to see if Nancy knows where we can rent a walker." I wanted to get one for her before she changed her mind.

"Okay," she answered casually and opened her snack pack of chicken, nuts, and raisins.

Nancy gave me directions to a medical supply store nearby, where we rented one for ten dollars a week. We did not expect her to need the walker for a long period, confident that she would soon be better.

In spite of her earlier objections, Sybil found that she enjoyed the walker because of the convenience of certain freedoms it allowed her. She would lift her numb right hand onto the bar with her left; and then, with the primary weight on her left side, she was able to rise from both the recliner at the clinic and the bed at the motel. The feeling of more independence gave her a boost of enthusiasm.

We found a cafeteria where Sybil could walk through the line on her own and select food at her own pace. I slid her tray for her while she made her choices. She was further relieved when no one here stared at her. We saw a couple of other diners with walkers like hers. A thoughtful waiter lifted her tray and took it to a table for her. She flashed him a beautiful smile when she thanked him.

The second night after we moved into our "upgraded suite," a boisterous group of construction workers coming in off their evening shift awakened us at midnight. It was obvious that they wanted to enjoy beer and banter with their friends outside their rooms. They seemed to be in no hurry to quiet down or go inside their rooms. There was no way either of us could sleep unless they left the parking lot to go to their separate rooms. The next morning Randy complained to the management. But that night it was the same loud midnight performance.

The incident strengthened our resolve to find other living arrangements. Sybil needed sleep if she was to heal. And we all needed the rest to relieve our stress. The motel had served a good purpose as a stopover, but we would have to move on.

Ideal Lodging Discovered

*The best setting for Sybil: cozy
lodging, peaceful surroundings*

I stepped up my search the following day; and, after eliminating
several options, I discovered a trailer park that was much nearer
the clinic and seemed as if it might have some rentals. We drove
to the area after Sybil and Randy finished the day's treatment. The
area was clean and nicely landscaped. Randy parked the car near
the entrance and went to the office; finding it locked, he walked
across the street to knock on the door of a resident. The woman
who answered his query told him that the property owner would
not be in until the next day.

As we waited for Randy, Sybil was sitting silently in the back
and did not speak until he returned to the car. Then she presented
an idea to us.

"Jim and Sherry have a camper," she suggested. "I know that
they would let us use it."

"Is that the one they use at the Gun Club?" I asked. The Gun
Club has big weekend events for target practice in rural Rutherford
County. Bill and Jim did most of the cooking for the weekend
events, and they used Jim's motor home to store supplies.

She nodded.

"I remember seeing the camper there, but I didn't go inside. Is there enough sleeping room for us?"

"There's bound to be. They take the family camping in it, so I am sure there is room enough for the three of us."

"I've been inside it," Randy said, "and there is plenty of room. Bill could drive it down for us."

Sybil saved her voice for significant conversations on the telephone. This was one of those important times. She asked Bill about using Jim and Sherry's camper. "He is sure that we can use it," she reported after talking with Bill. "They'll drive it down, probably this weekend." She looked at me and smiled. "It's just what we need. Now, Mom, it's up to you to find us a good campground."

"Awesome responsibility," I laughed, "but I can do it. I'll search during your treatments."

We were excited. Another prayer for Sybil had been answered. Everyone was with us, and events were going our way. We celebrated with another meal from Siam Garden Thai.

Bill called later that same day. Jim and Sherry were delighted to be able to do something for Sybil. Without hesitation, Jim made immediate plans to drive down with Bill. Kenny generously agreed to fly down to St. Petersburg to take them back to North Carolina after they delivered the motor home.

I set about finding a place to park our new home. There were an amazing number of sites to choose from. After eliminating or being eliminated from several motor home parks, one impressed me enough to take Sybil there for her approval and Randy for advice.

Holiday Campground in Seminole sounded like the perfect place. It was located just across the road from Lake Seminole Park, a designated wildlife habitat and sanctuary where raccoons, alligators, waterfowl, hawks, bald eagles, black vultures, tortoises, turtles, and snakes reside. It has grills, picnic tables, a playground, water fountains, and restrooms. A two-mile trail winds through the 250-acre park.

Behind the campground side, there is river where occupants

can fish. I thought Randy would like fishing there, but his real love was the challenge of fishing in the ocean, not from a riverbank. With the river in back and the park in front, the campsite was distinctly more comfortable than campgrounds simply bordered with asphalt. It also seemed cleaner.

On the property was a tiny post office, a swimming pool, playground, bathhouses, laundry, and a clubhouse used for chapel and other activities posted during the week; such as games, dances and crafts. There were far more activities than we would be able to take part in, but the idea was appealing. We all felt that Sybil would improve and possibly be able to participate in some of the fun activities later. The post office and Internet hookup could keep us connected for daily comfort, and there was a cable hookup so that Sybil could watch television.

Randy drove us to see the campground. He and Sybil waited while I went into the office to see about arrangements for a rental spot. There were two women behind the counter, both busy scribbling on large columned sheets. The heavier of the two, a young brown-haired woman, was the one I had spoken with earlier by phone. She had a spot selected for us and gave me directions so that we could look it over before deciding to make a deposit. The vacancy was four streets past the entrance.

We watched for the numbers, some barely visible. Then Randy pointed to a grassy space with a small tree beside the parking spot. "There it is."

"Look, Sybil, you have a lemon tree!" I saw yellow fruit sprinkled among the limbs of a small tree on the lot.

"Lemonade," she smiled.

The river was just across the street. The surrounding trailers sat in well-manicured spaces, some with flowers and other creative landscaping features. It was an Eden compared to the aging Grant Hotel. We could hardly contain our excitement as we drove back to the office so I could put down a deposit and officially make us "happy campers."

Sybil had been doing especially well with her walker, skillfully maneuvering the short step up from the motel parking space. The steps on the motor home, however, would be a different matter. They were spaced too far apart, and the opening was too narrow for her to manage with her walker. We all realized the nuisance and discussed our options.

Sybil came up with the solution. "Bill can build an access ramp and bring it with them when they come." Later, when she mentioned the subject during their evening call, he agreed.

We anxiously awaited Bill's call on the day that he and Jim drove into town. Bill never saw our "grand ole" Grant Motel. Instead, they drove directly to the campground. When the call came, however, we discovered that our campsite would be different from our original choice, something having to do with the type of motor coach. I never understood the reasoning.

"Uh-oh, Sybil," I said when I heard, "there goes your lemon tree." She smiled and shrugged her shoulders.

I was happy to go check out of the motel while Sybil and Randy waited patiently in the car. While I stood at the front desk to take my leave, Mary and the motel owner asked me about Sybil. They were also interested in knowing more about Joe's clinic. I gave them a brief summary about Albarin. They gave me their personal phone numbers and asked that I let them know about Sybil from time to time.

It was with relief that I handed Mary the TV remote and the telephone with the frazzled cord. We drove away, excited about having a new and more comfortable home away from home.

Randy is very observant. We had barely reached the campground gate when he pointed to our right, "There's Bill," he said. We saw Bill waving his arms, standing beside a camper two rows over, within sight of the entrance and camp store. I was pleased with the new location. We would be able to scurry swiftly from our parking space to the post office, laundry, and community showers. This was a special advantage for the periods when there might be only one person with Sybil.

Jim and Bill had quickly set up camp. A green rug stretched

across the grass underneath a canopy cover to create a "patio." The men had set lawn chairs in a semicircle facing the door.

After cheerful hugs and handshakes, we settled into the chairs, everyone talking at once. Bill and Jim amused us with their description of the trip from North Carolina. "We were running about eight-five miles an hour," Bill said. "Moreover, everything was working perfect for us. Nobody got in our way, and every time we pulled into the passing lane, everybody would move over. Jim said to me, 'This is an act of God. It's gotta' be. Because we've got this thing floor boarded down all the way, the pedal to the metal, and everybody's getting out of our way. This is an act of God.'"

I slipped silently away to see the inside of the camper. The cozy motor home was just what Sybil needed. The interior walls were within arm's reach of just about everything, so she could hold on to them and maneuver about without help.

When I saw the tiny shower stall with a handheld shower sprayer, I called out "The shower is built just for you, Sybil. It's really small, and you can sit on a corner seat to bathe and shampoo." Only a step away on the opposite side was small sink and a commode. The sliding door to the bed was between the shower and sink, and just one step in the opposite direction was the kitchen beside the exterior door.

On the other side of the entrance, a beige sleeper sofa sat against a wall, opposite a small table with chairs. Cabinets were overhead on both sides. Up front, there was a bunk bed above the driver and passenger seats, and between the seats was a television set. Sybil would be able to see the TV from the sofa or the table. That was good. The kitchen held staples, condiments, and cleaning supplies. Sherry had put a package of bed and bath goodies inside a small clothes closet.

I thanked Jim profusely. "This is absolutely perfect! We are all so grateful to you, Jim."

"You are more than welcome, Iris. We're just happy that we can do something to help. And if we can do anything else, all you have to do is ask."

Jim led Randy around the motor van explaining the technical hookups for electricity, gas, plumbing, and cable. I relied on Randy to take care of those things while I tended to the exploration of the women's territory inside.

Their mission accomplished, Randy drove Jim and Bill to meet Kenny at the airport for their homeward flight. The new arrangement was perfect. Unfortunately, the handicap ramp Bill made to fit the motor home door was too small for Sybil to use her walker on. In addition, it was too heavy for me to set in place. I did not have the strength to lift it. I would have to help Sybil maneuver the two steep steps. She and I disagreed on which foot to put forward first. Since neither was easy, she just did the best she could as I held her.

Sybil and I were happy as kids in a new playhouse. We explored every inch of our bright new lodging. At this point, she did not need the walker inside the motor home. She walked along the aisle easily as she held onto the kitchen counter, occasionally balancing herself. She was beaming as she made her way between the shower and commode stalls to the bed at the end; then, still smiling broadly, she walked back through the full length of the home to the TV set.

It was a thrill to see her moving so easily by herself, seemingly healthy and certainly proud to be on her own here.

She turned the knob on the television set, but the channels were fuzzy. Her smile faded as she turned to me, "It's not working."

I went to the set and looked at the back for an adjustment. "Looks like we're not connected to cable, yet," I said, "but it is included with our rent. I'll run over to the office to report it."

At the door, I told her, "I'll be right back. Meanwhile, don't go anywhere."

She looked at her walker and laughed. "Like I could fly away on this piece of tin."

Even though I rushed back from the office, the maintenance man beat me to the camper, and within a matter of minutes he had the set working and with a good clear picture. This was a good example of the prompt attention the campground management gave during our entire stay.

When Sybil maneuvered over to adjust the controls, she looked at me and laughed, "Maybe we should've brought the remote from the motel."

I laughed with her. "The remote and telephone were ransom I had to pay to get us out of there. Part of the check-in, check-out process. Just like turning in the key." It was plain to see that we were quite happy with our new surroundings. "We'll find you a remote tomorrow."

"No problem. It looks like we've got everything else we need right here."

Sybil had mastered the art of bathing with only her left hand, and the tiny shower seemed custom made for this situation. The seat allowed her to relax and take her time. She was able to cautiously shave both her legs smooth and shampoo her hair with her left hand. I admired her patience. Meanwhile, I laid a towel across the bed for her to sit on to dry, and I put fresh clothes beside it. When she finished, she twirled herself out of the shower, into the bedroom, and onto her bed with the help of the facing wall, seemingly without effort. Only then did she call for me to help her with her clothes. She could slip into some of her clothes on her own, depending on the garment, but with some she needed my help. She was so happy to have the convenience of the small area that allowed her a larger measure of independence.

Before daylight on the first morning in our new quarters, Randy eased down from the high bunk bed, where he had slept, onto a chair piled with extra cushions that he used as a stepladder to reach the height of the cot. Then he slipped out the door to go to the community shower building nearby. While he was gone, I dressed and restored my sleeper to a sofa before starting breakfast.

Waking Sybil was not a problem now. When she was a teen, I would wake her up and have a conversation with her, but when I left the room, she would often fall back into a deep sleep and then not remember what we had said earlier. Now she heard me moving about and swung herself around the wall into the little bathroom. She was too excited about getting to her daily treatments to stay in bed late.

Late Tuesday evening, Randy noticed a smell like something burning in the camper. That was disconcerting, of course, so I called the campground office. They recommended Art's RV Service in Largo. Art Sarrach was not in the mood to come out that late in the day, but I begged.

"If we smell smoke, it could become a fire, and my daughter is paralyzed on one side and cannot move without help. There is no way we'll be able to sleep tonight if we can't find out what is wrong."

Thankfully, he gave in and came right away. Afterward Art agreed that it would have been very dangerous if he had not come to replace a heater board. He took note of Sybil languishing helplessly on the sofa. He sympathized and told me that he was glad he came and would come again right away if we had problems with anything else in the home. I felt that it was unnecessary to tell Sybil that we paid him three hundred dollars to make the repair.

Dr. Joe had been telling us that as Sybil began to heal, she would feel pain. But until now, her pain had been minimal. One morning, shortly after Randy's return from his shower, Sybil put a naked leg out from the side of the bedroom door panel. "Ta dah!" she cried and thrust her arm into the air like a stripper show. And with sparkling eyes and a huge smile, she declared excitedly, "I've got pain!"

Randy and I laughed happily at her dramatic performance and thoughts of what it might mean.

"Where is your pain?" I asked.

She proudly pointed to her right leg. Her broad smile spoke of her delight and expectation that the pain was indeed a good sign.

"You've got feeling in your *right* leg?" Randy asked.

When she nodded, Randy and I smiled at each other. We, too, saw this as a good sign.

While her mood was high, Sybil decided it was time for a haircut. Indeed, it was time for both of us. Our hair styling days had always been outings that invariably included either lunch or dinner and a glass of wine. We had fond memories of those happy days.

I referred to the yellow pages for a beauty parlor close to us and found one just across the river in the Seminole Mall, Rendezvous Beauty Salon. It would be convenient, and one strange salon would be no different to us from another strange beauty parlor. When I called for the appointment, I emphasized promptness so that Sybil would not have to wait. The woman gave me her assurances and offered me two ten o'clock appointments for the following morning.

Randy let us out at the curb in front of the shop and then left to do some shopping on his own. The thoughtful proprietor was watching for us and promptly escorted Sybil to a chair. After I waited a few minutes longer for my turn, a friendly Hispanic woman ushered me to the shampoo sink. The delay created a short wait for Sybil, but she looked lovely and managed her walker beautifully on her way to a waiting chair.

While Sybil sat patiently, an elderly woman maneuvered a walker to sit beside her. Sybil was delighted. She and her new friend exchanged "walker stories" while the woman waited for her appointment. When I approached the front area, I saw another woman speaking to Sybil as she rose to her feet with the help of her walker.

"What happened to you?" the tall haughty woman asked bluntly.

Sybil announced brightly cheerful and slightly sarcastic, "I've got a brain tumor!"

The woman's furrowed expression changed to one of uncomfortable frustration.

"Oh," was all she could manage in response as she turned abruptly toward the exit.

Sybil laughed about the incident while we waited at the door for Randy. We were still laughing when he drove up. We could laugh easily because we felt sure that Sybil's tumor was temporary. We were having our happiest week yet in St. Petersburg.

On Sunday morning Randy, Sybil, and I joined the other campers in the clubhouse for a chapel service. Worshipers seated in portable metal chairs filled the huge hall. A pleasant elderly usher welcomed us. He and another man hastily gathered three folded chairs and helped Randy place them near the door. We did not know whether Sybil would be able to sit through the entire worship service. She maneuvered the walker easily now and took her seat between Randy and me. We were grateful for our good fortune thus far and happy to thank God for it.

The following afternoon, Sybil looked down at the sandals on her feet. "I'd like to have another pair like these," she said. She was wearing a pair of beige cloth sandals. "They are so comfortable." I was glad she wanted something for herself.

Before she changed her mind, I left her with Randy and drove over to the Seminole Mall. I was surprised to find the exact style of shoe at Beal's department store. I bought her a soft green color. Her pants had been getting tighter, so I also bought her a knit shirt and short set a size larger than what she was wearing. She was delighted that I had found the shoes she had asked for.

Neither of us thought that the swelling in her stomach was anything other than ordinary weight gain. She had not had her monthly period yet, but we never thought about it. She and I were relieved that she did not have to be bothered with the nuisance of it just now.

Sybil's pain was now becoming more severe. She was still taking dexamethasone for brain swelling, Xanax for anxiety, and MGN3, a supplement that Joe had recommended. But she was not taking anything for pain.

I made it a point to talk with Dr. Mayer, who prescribed Percocet, one tablet every six hours as needed.

"How is Sybil doing?" I asked.

"Where do you go to church?" he asked. It was a disquieting response to my question. I felt a chill.

"We've been going to the chapel at the campground where we are living," I replied shakily. He seemed to be saying that prayer is all we have. I did not want to hear that implication.

A couple of years later, when I was prepared to hear him answer, I asked Dr. Mayer about his peculiar response. He admitted, "Uh, well, I guess indirectly I was saying that. Having been a preacher before I was a doctor, it was sort of ingrained in me, and I just ask that question or one similar to it. I don't usually ask where you go to church. I usually ask what your spiritual resources are. Some people ask, 'Your what?' I think that ought to be part of medical practice. After all, He who made us certainly must know how to keep us put together or correct what's wrong with us. I also just wish people in the medical profession would be more conscious in offering hope to people. In my opinion, one problem with the medical community is that many doctors do not have an open mind about alternative medications. And if you don't have an open mind, you can't teach anybody anything."

But during our time at the clinic, I refused to think about Dr. Mayer's question. Sybil, Randy, and I were optimistic and wanted to keep it that way. Hope was our refuge and strength.

Then Randy broke the sad news to us that it was necessary for him to leave. He had two construction jobs in progress, Richard's cabin in Blowing Rock, North Carolina, and a friend's project on an island near Spring Creek, Florida. He was a pillar of strength, and we were so grateful that that he had been with us during the initial days of this intense experience. I wanted to go away alone to cry. We would feel the loss. Reluctantly, we contacted Jayne to search Priceline on the Internet for a one-way flight to Charlotte.

Randy's announcement coincided with a change at the clinic. The new schedule of therapy would alternate weeks between the St. Petersburg location and an existing chelation treatment center in Tampa, where Joe currently administered therapy several days a week. It would be a longer, less comfortable trip for Sybil, but she was a trooper and accepted the change cheerfully as a new adventure.

Jayne scheduled an airline ticket for Randy to leave from Tampa the morning before our first scheduled treatment in Tampa. Sybil wanted to treat him to a farewell dinner at his favorite restaurant, Carrabba's Italian Grill. It was just down the street from our health food store, Richard's Whole Foods, where we stopped on the way. While at Richard's, an attractive young woman with a healthy tan and athletic body spoke to me.

She asked abruptly, gesturing in Randy's direction, "Is he your husband?"

Randy is a handsome friendly man and former model who has on more than one occasion been approached by girls and women interested in getting to know him.

"Oh, no, he is my son."

She was obviously relieved by my answer. "I don't usually do this, but ..." she began boldly, and then she proceeded to give me a full profile of herself. After handing me her business card and asking me to give it to him, she disappeared behind the vitamin counter, where she overheard Randy tell the familiar cashier that we were on our way to have dinner at Carrabba's.

When we drove into the parking lot, we saw a line of waiting diners stretched along the sidewalk in front of the door.

"Oh, no," Sybil moaned.

"Do you want Randy to see how long the wait is? Maybe we can wait in the car."

"No, I want to go home," she stated emphatically.

"Randy, why don't you take us home and come back here for take-out?" I suggested. He agreed. Nevertheless, I was so disappointed for her. I had been hoping she would enjoy the night out.

When Randy returned to the restaurant alone, he went to Carrabba's bar to have a beer and order our food. Just as he sat on a barstool, the bartender approached him with a cordless phone in hand. "Are you Randy?" He nodded and the server handed him the phone. He took the call, apprehensive about Sybil, only to discover it was the stranger from Richard's. The girl asked if she could join him there for dinner. He politely excused himself by telling her that he was only there to pick up take-out. And when pressed for another date, he told her that he was to fly to North Carolina the following day. And then, just as he handed the phone back to the bartender, another unfamiliar young woman sat down on the stool next to him. "May I buy you another beer?" she asked.

"No, thank you. I don't have time for another. I am just picking up an order for my mother and sister. They are waiting for me."

"Oh," she said, disappointed.

The waiter handed him the large to-go package. "Thanks anyway," he told her as he left his seat.

Sybil was cheerful at dinner and much more relaxed than she would have been in a crowd. We teased Randy about the sudden attention from groupies.

"You're leaving too soon, Randy," Sybil said. "Just when you're getting some action here." The Florida belles were just now discovering him. It was a bittersweet evening and the last one that the three of us would share for a while.

We left early for the airport so that Randy could help us find the new clinic. The Howard Frankland Bridge alone stretches for almost five miles over Tampa Bay. The drive across the waterway is very beautiful and not as intimidating as it sounds, because it does not soar as high above the water as I had expected.

We watched for a small shopping mall named Carrollwood Center on the left.

"There's the 'big red-hot,'" said Randy. He and I spotted the huge sign on the roof of a small building on the inside corner of the strip mall. The clinic is beside Abby's Health Food Store, and Starbucks Coffee is in the same block of shops.

It was a fun ride, with the three of us laughing and talking as usual, but Sybil and I fought back tears when we left Randy at the airport gate. It was depressing to see him lift his luggage and disappear behind the door. Sybil and I had a quiet, thoughtful drive back across the bay without him.

We were not alone for long, however. Bill soon drove in for a weekend. As I was helping Sybil fasten her bra the morning after he arrived, she said pathetically, "I think I could fasten it myself, but I forgot how." She saw it as another brain malfunction.

"That's not surprising," I said. "A brassiere is a complicated contraption. It is not easy for me to remember, even with two hands. Sometimes I start on the wrong side." It is confusing to fasten it in the front upside down, slide the fastened side to the back, raise the cups right side up, and then pull the straps over the arms one at a time. I well understood Sybil's frustration.

"It's a hell of a lot harder than learning to tie your shoes." Sybil laughed. "Men have no clue. They only know how to take a bra off." Then she observed, "I think I need a larger size."

I agreed. "It looks like you do. Why don't we go get you a couple of larger ones today?"

Surprisingly, she wanted to go, so the three of us went shopping at Target. Bill went into the store ahead of us to get a motorized chair. It did not take her any time to learn how to speed away from us through the store.

It was such a pleasure to walk with Sybil while she shopped. That is all I had to do. She maneuvered the wheelchair with ease as she and I went to the women's lingerie department while Bill browsed over in hardware. For that short time, she seemed unaware of her disability. We laughed as she steered within inches of products that were hanging on the shelves, but she never hit anything. She was more confident than I was about her agility.

Despite the fun and the ease of using the wheelchair, Sybil declared a firm no to our suggestion that we rent one for her to use full time.

On Sunday, the three of us went to camp church. The ushers quickly got three seats and unfolded them for us.

This is the e-mail message we sent out that evening: "Bill is in St. Petersburg, Florida. He arrived a few hours after Randy left us on Friday. He will be with us until Tuesday. We had a great day with him teaching Sybil to drive a motorized wheel chair at Target. She had only two bump-ups and no casualties. Bill's toe will be okay, eventually. Progress continues well. She still needs to rest daily, but she's gathering strength and is more active during the day. Randy had to go back to NC. We enjoyed having him here and could not have managed without him during the first trying weeks. He knows we're better equipped to continue without him now. We are still encouraged by all your continued support. Love and gratitude to all, Iris and Sybil."

On Monday, Bill drove us to Seminole to an Einstein Bagel shop we had located in a small shopping area there. We picked up breakfast bagels to eat on our way to Tampa. When we reached the clinic at Carrollwood, Bill parked the car in front of the door and waited while we got out of the car and Sybil maneuvered her walker to the building. Bill drove away to park while she and I explored the new treatment center.

The patient's area was discouraging. There were no recliners here. Instead, there were low-slung chairs with a seamless contour seat that hugged the body. The style is very comfortable, but it is extremely difficult to get out of, even for a healthy person. The seats are too near the floor to rise up without a struggle. I once owned one like that myself and discovered that rolling out from the side was the simplest way to get up from floor level. I happily gave mine away. *Bill could help Sybil out of one today, but what about next time?*

I helped ease Sybil into one of the chairs next to the door, put a pillow behind her back, and gave her a blanket. She sat low enough for me to put her snack bag on the floor within reach. Joe and Jann Ramsey, a nurse we had not seen before, were measuring the formula. Sybil was comfortable and waiting patiently for her injection when Bill came into the room. He stayed in the room with her during treatment. (In hindsight, I regret not staying in the treatment room with her more often during the process. Most of the time I ran errands instead. This is something I would have done differently.)

I took the opportunity to go to Abbey's, where I browsed through a special selection of books, magazines and pamphlets on health, searching for more help with Sybil's condition. I found spelt flour and pasta, a bagful of assorted nuts for Sybil's pack, and a prepared vegetarian salad to go with our evening meal.

Bill was ready to leave early Tuesday morning. He planned to head east to I-95, a route to Frances Marion College in Florence, South Carolina, where he would watch son David play baseball. Then David would ride back home with his dad after the game.

I waited outside the camper while he and Sybil said good-bye. We were ready to go to the St. Petersburg clinic after his departure. Before he left, he came to the door and spoke to me. "Come here, Iris, and show me how you can take care of Sybil after I leave."

She was standing at the door waiting for me to help her down the steps. As I held her while she stepped gingerly off the two high steps, one step at a time, I wondered, *What did he think I had been doing during the weeks before he came?* I handed her the walker that was leaning against the side of the trailer. She stood with help of the walker as he went to his car and drove away.

When Sybil and I were alone, we found it was rather comfortable to relax and not be responsible for anyone else. We managed very well. I took care of buying groceries while she was in treatment. As for the laundry, I ran back and forth from the camp laundry center. First I would put the loads in and leave them to wash while I went back to be with Sybil. Then I would rush over and put them in the dryer. On my last trip, I would grab them out of the dryer and then run back to be with Sybil while I folded and pressed.

When some of the machines were out of order, I could not always find an empty washer or dryer and would have to wait, checking back and forth between our campsite and the laundry. Thankfully, another camper told me about a private laundromat in another location. It was one with an attendant on duty all the time and was less than a mile from the camp. Even though I would have to drive there, I could leave the laundry in the attendant's care and only needed to make two quick trips.

After the Target shopping trip and Sybil's experience of freedom with a wheelchair, Bill and I suggested that we rent one for her to use. Sybil's rejection of the wheelchair was similar to her delayed decision on the walker. We shelved the idea for the time being. It was understandable. Giving in to a crutch of any sort meant giving up more independence, not to mention drawing more stares. Even though Sybil had walked into the clinic her first day with the minimal assistance of our two hands and then later with the walker, I never saw those declines as a worsening of her situation. Rather, I felt that the painful feeling in her right foot was a good thing, because there was now feeling where previously it had been numb. I also wondered if some of the loss of strength in the right arm and leg could be from long unused muscles. She and I talked about that.

I spoke to Dr. Joe and Dr. Mayer, and they encouraged me to devise an exercise program of some sort. Joe suggested that we use one of the machines in his gym room at the clinic. She could lie on her back, and the machine itself would work her legs similar to a bicycle ride.

"It may build up strength in your leg. And Joe said that we could adjust the speed," I coaxed her.

"The only exercise I want to do is to press the TV remote," she said laughing.

"Okay, we'll take it easy, just a few minutes to start with. I'll do the treadmill while you do the leg thing."

On Friday, Sybil was able to walk into the gym holding my arm. We met a woman whom we had been seen occasionally in passing as she patronized the gym. "You are doing really well," she told Sybil, noticing that she was not using the walker.

"Yes, I'm doing great!" Sybil answered cheerfully.

Well, that success was short-lived. First of all, there was no attendant, so we had to figure out how the machine worked all on our own. I helped Sybil onto the contraption, settling each of her legs over a hump that held her knees in a bent position. "Is this okay?" I asked. She was lying down, sporting a doubtful look on her face.

"I'm too far down," she said.

I reached under her shoulders to scoot her further backward toward the end. "Okay, how's that?"

"Good," she replied. "Now what?"

I saw an on button between some other controls and switched the machine on.

"Whoa!" Sybil called out immediately. "Whoa!"

"What?" I switched the button off instantly.

"It's too fast! Get me out of here!"

"Well, you're already there, so let me just see if I can slow it down with these other controls. Joe said this would be good for you."

She relented reluctantly.

I twisted what appeared to be a speed knob and hesitantly turned the on switch again while keeping my hand ready to turn it off right away if needed. The machine started more slowly. "How's that?" I asked.

"Better, but not good," she answered.

"I'll get you off in five minutes."

In less than three, she wanted off. As I helped her off the exerciser, I could tell that she was less able to walk than she had been when she got on. It had been a mistake to bring her. I wanted to do the best of everything I could for her, but this idea was not good.

"I'm so sorry."

"It's okay this time, Mom, but I'm not going to do that again," she said kindly but firmly.

During our second trip to the Tampa clinic, I took Sybil to the treatment room and again tucked her into one of the low-slung seats. I put her walker near the door out of the way. She was able to use it in St. Petersburg where the recliners were high enough for her to grasp it, but not here in these chairs. She smiled at me, and then opened her book. The other patients, some of whom she had not met in St. Petersburg, were talking softly among themselves.

I went outside where there was a sidewalk umbrella table near the clinic entrance. The weather was beautiful in Florida this time of year. I had barely taken my seat, when Jann, the nurse, opened the door and called out to me.

"Sybil needs to use the bathroom," she said.

I rushed inside to help her. I set the walker beside me and took her hands to raise her up, but she was too far down and was dead weight. I was afraid I would pull her arms out of their sockets. I felt so helpless.

Jann spoke sharply from behind me. "Wait! That is not the way. Let me show you how to do this." I wondered why Jann had not helped her to the bathroom in the first place instead of wasting time finding me. It was obvious that Sybil was in a hurry. She had a pained look on her face, but said nothing when Jann put her arms all the way under Sybil's arms and lifted her easily upward. As I slid the walker in front of her, I saw her stained pants and wanted to cry for her. I snatched her blanket to cover her from behind as we moved unsteadily out of the room. Thereafter, Sybil wore sanitary pads for protection from another such accident.

Cushing's Syndrome
Sybil falls subject to an unexpected condition

We were in Tampa, and Dr. Mayer was having one of his regular private talks with Sybil. I walked in just as he concluded with the words "moon face," which is a symptom of exogenous Cushing's syndrome. The syndrome was a side effect of dexamethasone, the medication that controlled the swelling in her brain.

After Dr. Mayer's words, I noticed for the first time that her face had changed to a swollen appearance, full and round. It happened so gradually that I had not realized it before. Now that the doctor suggested it, it was obvious. I could not believe I had missed the drastic change.

When I learned more about it from research, I realized that there were other signs we had not recognized. Her menstrual period had stopped, her neck had become fat, and her stomach was swollen (central obesity); her weakness and fatigue were also symptoms.

Sybil had evidently noticed changes, but she and I did not discuss the physical differences, just the cause and effect. I did not want her to feel that I thought her body was changing abnormally.

Dr. Mayer's observation set Sybil to worrying about taking the dexamethasone. Now that she had become self-conscious about her moon face, the most noticeable feature of the disease, she asked whether she could go off the drug. He told her that she could taper off gradually. We did not realize it was a catch-22. When she tapered off, the swelling in her brain would increase, as would the pain. In retrospect, I realize that the compassionate doctor wanted to make her as happy as he could and knew that only a miracle could save her. But unlike the blunt oncologist back in Spartanburg, he was being thoughtful and kind.

Meanwhile, we talked about a physical therapist to help with her arm and leg. On our shopping trip to Target, Bill had bought a bungee cord, which he attached to a cabinet doorknob above the sofa for Sybil to exercise her arm. But she was not able to use it. She could not reach it alone, and when I handed it to her, the tension was too strong for her to handle. She was naturally skeptical about physical therapy after my unfortunate mistake at the gym.

"I'll ask Joe to recommend a good therapist, and we'll just make an appointment to simply talk about it before anyone touches you. Okay?"

Joe did not know of anyone, so I went to the old standby, the Yellow Pages. "Sports Massage Therapist and Personal Trainer, Travis Skaggs. 5610 Fourth Street North." That was just down the street from Grant Motel. "Athletic injury recovery, backache relief, deep tissue massage, headache relief, neuromuscular therapy, pain management, shiatsu/acupressure, and relaxation massage." The last four listings sounded promising.

Travis was a lean, short, leather-tanned man, whose smile was just a slight spread of his lips with his mouth closed. He was proud of his credentials, but it was not comfortable to talk with him. I did not know whether he was skeptical about working with Sybil because of her cancer or felt that his therapy was just what she needed. At any rate, he cautiously demonstrated the therapy himself by using weights for his arms and legs. Sybil and I both cringed. It would be far too much for her.

Neither Sybil nor I were impressed. This was not an ill reflection on Mr. Skaggs. Sometimes the chemistry is simply not there. I also was afraid that he would hurt rather than help. Nonetheless, I was disappointed as usual when the promise of additional healing failed.

"I'm not going to take treatment from him," Sybil stated as we left the building.

"Good," I said, "I don't feel comfortable with him, either. We can just wait until we get back to North Carolina. Maybe we can do our water exercises again. Those are low impact, and you like them, probably more than any other exercise you have done, other than swimming."

She nodded in agreement. Because her voice would weaken, Sybil and I could not engage in long conversations. It was always stronger in the morning but gradually weakened during the day. We often made one-liner quips and developed our own sort of sign language for some things.

Occasionally it would be difficult for Sybil to grasp a word that she wanted to use. Something would come out incorrectly, and she knew immediately that it came out wrong; or a word she wanted to use would not come to her at all. She would shake her head in exasperation and say, "Misfired again." She never wanted me to fill in the word for her so that she could try on her own to remember and use it. When her first thought misfired, I would wait for her to think for herself until it came to her. It was always tempting to prompt her, but given enough time, she could usually summon the word.

"You still remember a lot of things better than I do, and I don't have a brain tumor for an excuse," I would tell her. She would just look at me with a wry smile.

It was becoming more of a struggle for Sybil to use the walker. She was tiring faster, and her right foot tended to turn inward more often. She had to move very slowly to keep her feet straight. Finally when the foot flopped with her once too often, she stared at it angrily, "S——!"

"Sybil," I started hesitantly, "I think that it would make moving around much easier if you would let me get you a wheelchair."

This time, much to my surprise, she agreed readily. I prepared to get her one before she changed her mind. We got her in and out of the bathroom before I left. I made sure she was comfortable on the sofa with her book, remote, and snack, everything in reach. Then I drove directly across the river to Arden's Medical Supply in Seminole. I knew where the medical equipment store was located in the Seminole Mall because I had seen it when I bought Sybil's sandals. Unbeknownst to Sybil, I had gone in to inquire about the cost of a wheelchair. It would be twenty-five dollars a week.

I went directly to the checkout counter and asked the salesperson there to see the smaller wheelchairs. Together we selected a standard user-friendly chair. The clerk at Arden promised to send someone to the parking lot to help me load the chair that I had rolled out of the store, but no one showed up. It was up to me to find a way to put the awkward load into the trunk. It was terribly confusing. I was nearly in tears when I finally figured it out. Even so, it was necessary to use a bungee cord, because the trunk would not close all the way.

Transition

I did not recognize this new phase
as negative progress

The chair proved to be a blessing for both of us, especially getting in and out of the recliners at the St. Petersburg clinic. Sybil could easily twist around into the wheelchair. We could move her much faster, especially through the halls at the clinics, and she could wheel into the handicapped bathroom stalls. The motor home was the only place we could not use it, but she could still move through there by holding onto the cabinets.

We soon discovered that Sybil was much more comfortable remaining in her wheelchair during treatment. It eliminated the aggravation of trying to get in and out of those "on the floor" chairs in Tampa. I easily rolled her in and out of the clinic. She adjusted really well to the new chair and was happy with the extra freedom it offered; she could now move without fear of her right foot twisting, as long as it sat on the foot pedal.

In late February, we had a pleasant surprise. My long-time friend, Joan Strom, drove down from Lake Lure, North Carolina. When she later spoke of the visit, Joan said, "I just wanted to come and cook. I love to cook. We had Thai food and lots of fresh fruit, and Sybil knew she could not have sugar. I was just amazed at her sense of humor. We laughed a lot. It wasn't a pity party."

The evening she arrived, Joan gave Sybil a pedicure, and I gave her a manicure. Joan had one of Sybil's feet in her hands working on the pedicure when Jayne called from North Carolina. I handed the phone to Sybil.

Jayne said that she and Sandra Dexter were together reminiscing about Sybil and some of their good times together. "One of the funny things we just remembered about you," she told Sybil, "is that you never let anyone touch your feet."

Sybil, surprised by that memory, looked at the foot Joan held in her hand and laughed. "Then there is no way you can guess what I am doing right now." She smiled broadly at Joan, who was painting her toenails. "Joan Strom is giving me a pedicure." She laughed again, when Jayne replied, "I don't believe you."

Sybil was able to style her hair and put on makeup without assistance. In fact, she was doing a great job with her good left side. But she could not do her nails, so the pedicure and manicure were a real treat for her, for she had always kept her nails looking pretty.

Joan later recalled Sybil's independence. "The motor home was kind of a neat little place. Everything was close so that she could get up. She could get to the bathroom. Boy, she loved her showers. She always looked so fresh, smelled so good, and seemed so high. I marvel at that, I do."

As a part of her visit, Joan planned to sign up for chelation as treatment for her heart condition, arrhythmia. She drove with us to Tampa so that she could start the therapy. Chelation was the reason for the symbol of the big heart on Joe's signs.

When we arrived at the clinic, Joe, Georgiana, and Jean were not there. There had been a wreck on Gandy Bridge just before they crossed it, and they were stopped on the bridge in the traffic.

Dr. Mayer and Jann were doing what they could in the treatment room, which was filling fast with clients. I wheeled Sybil to an empty space and made sure she was comfortable with her book and snack pack beside her. Deedy was there and brought a tank of oxygen for her. Deedy looked after everyone, and I could rest assured that she would watch after Sybil.

When I went to the lobby, the phone was ringing, but there was no one to answer it. Joan could not sign up for her treatment until Georgiana came, so she went to the desk and started answering the telephone.

The small Tampa waiting room had mission style furniture, plain and straight legged. It was a stark contrast to the decor of the St. Petersburg clinic. Straight chairs lined two sides of the room. A corner table with magazines divided the seating. Everyone could hear each other in this room because of the close proximity between the chairs and desk.

I sat beside a nice-looking, middle-aged newcomer, Richard Jennings. He had been diagnosed with prostate cancer and had driven into town to investigate Dr. Joe's treatment. Joan was listening intently as she sat behind the desk to answer calls.

"How did you hear about Joe's clinic?" I asked him.

"A friend of mine in Texas told me about it. I just wanted to come check it out." He was skeptical about the benefits of the therapy.

When I realized that he was looking for a positive referral, I told him "you need to talk to a friend of ours, Pat McEwen. He is my son's best friend and the source of our original knowledge. He is very well informed, and he's the brother of a prostate cancer survivor, Jim McEwen. The traditional doctors wanted to operate, but Jim refused and came to Joe's clinic instead. Now he has no sign of cancer and just comes to the clinic for maintenance."

"I would like to talk to him," Richard said. "Do you have his number?"

"Sure. I know he would be glad to talk to you." I was looking in my purse for Pat's number when the telephone rang again.

I heard Joan say. "There is a traffic jam on the bridge due to an accident. He has been delayed. Oh, my God, Patrick, you're not going to believe this …"

"Is that our Pat?" I asked Joan.

She nodded. "… but there is someone here that wants to talk to you."

Richard and I looked at each other in surprise. "ESP" I said. "Looks like I don't have to find the number."

Joan held the telephone receiver up for Richard as he strode to the desk. It seemed to be a good sign for Richard, who had a long conversation with Pat and then an in-depth talk with Joan. By the time Joe and his staff arrived, Richard had made up his mind to sign up for Albarin treatments, and Joan would register for chelation. Since the patients had backed up waiting for Joe, Joan and Richard would begin the next day in St. Petersburg.

The following morning, Joan and Richard became better acquainted and decided to have lunch together. While Sybil sat with Joan and Richard for her twentieth treatment, Dr. Mayer wrote a prescription for an MRI. It was scheduled for the next day, a Friday.

I took Sybil back to the campground for her long afternoon nap. When she woke up, I settled her on the sofa to watch her TV programs, and then I drove over to Seminole for groceries. "Joan will probably be back here before I get back," I told her. It had been almost three hours since we left her at the clinic. I rushed through the grocery store to pick out the items on my list. When I left the parking lot, I remembered some pharmaceutical supplies that Sybil needed. Thinking that Joan would be with Sybil by now, I stopped by Walgreen's along my way home. It was a bad assumption, and now I regret that decision. Ordinarily, I would have made a second trip later so that Sybil would not be alone for such a long period.

When I drove through the campground gate, I saw immediately that Joan's van was not at our site. Right away I felt sick with guilt. I should not have stopped at the drugstore. It was even worse than I imagined. When I got to the camper door, I saw Sybil on the floor, halfway between the sofa and the counter. The counter should have been a prop for her, but she had fallen and could not get up. I was sick with remorse.

"Mom, where have you been?" she cried as tears streamed

down her distressed face. During her entire ordeal, I had not seen her so distraught. "I've got to go to the bathroom!"

"Oh, honey, I'm so sorry," I said as I tried to lift her off the floor. "I thought Joan would be back."

"I can't wait!" she cried.

"Hold on!" I said, and I leapt off the steps to retrieve the plastic tub we had used to soak her feet for the pedicure. I was able to scoot her over the floor to the top of the steps and set her feet on that first step so that I could hold her up. Bless her heart; she was able to empty her bladder standing up. We were both in tears when she finished. I felt so ashamed to have been responsible for her anguish.

By evening, Sybil and I had cheered up, and she was able to laugh about the incident. Joan brought dinner from a Thai Restaurant that she discovered on the way back from her delightful afternoon with Richard.

It was time for the anticipated and dreaded MRI. I stayed in the room with Sybil during the test. She joked with the nurses and asked me not to tell Bill about the test until we had the results. I promised that I would not. For some unknown reason, the person at the desk told me I could pick up the results on Saturday. I still do not know why they did not send them directly to Dr. Mayer.

Though I did not know how to interpret the pictures that I picked up on Saturday, there was a written report, and it mentioned something I did not want to acknowledge. All the discussions with doctors had been about tumors in her brain and lungs, but this report made a reference to tumors in her esophagus. I had a terrible sinking feeling. Fear gripped my heart. *Her fading voice*, I thought. It made sense that tumors in her throat would cause this. I said nothing about the written report to Sybil and Joan.

"We can't tell anything by these X-ray pictures," I told them. "We have to wait for Joe or Dr. Mayer to interpret these for us on Monday." And then I hid them away on a shelf overhead.

This was absolutely the worst weekend that I spent during our stay in St. Petersburg. The MRI result was constantly on my mind. Joan came down with arrhythmia and had to stay in bed. I was always nervous when she had arrhythmia and bed rest was all she could do for it. It was a double dose of helplessness.

I could not sleep, so I crept outside with a book. I sat near the door with an ear open for Sybil's call. I kept rereading the same page over and over, absorbing nothing. Then I prayed and tried desperately to clear my mind of terrifying thoughts.

Sybil's weekend e-mail message omitted any mention of the scan:

"Sybil Update—2/25/01. Still positive, but no big changes here. I would like to know what is going on in your neck of the woods, about children, animals, gossip, weather, and whatever. We do not get your news here. If you are not doing anything, tell us what your neighbors are doing. A special guest on board this week is our friend Joan Strom (just like Oprah, we have our own gourmet chef). She is preparing special 'healthy' meals for us. Love, Sybil."

On Monday, Joe discussed the test results with Sybil and me after she had had her treatment for that day. She sat listlessly in her wheelchair, her head drooping slightly. She was tired after therapy, as usual, but it was the first time I noticed that she had some trouble holding her head up.

Joe said that the large tumor on the left side of her brain had changed shape but had also reduced in size. The small one that was originally on the right side did not show up on this scan, indicating that it might be gone. He told us that he could not compare the lung results because the hospital in Spartanburg never sent the original report of her lungs. He did not mention the esophageal tumor, because he had no basis for comparison.

The Spartanburg clinic continued to ignore further requests for Sybil's lung X-rays. I consider their refusal to send pertinent information and tests an obstruction to Sybil's safety and well-being. Someone in Spartanburg had an opportunity to help Dr. Joe and Dr. Mayer in their fight to save Sybil. I do not know who was responsible for the hospital's denial, but it was an irresponsible act, whoever the guilty party or parties might be. It was as if the staff of Palmetto Hematology Oncology was saying, "If you will not come here, we will not help you."

I was disappointed, because the St. Petersburg scan seemed to show that there was a mass that should not be there. To me it appeared to be in her throat, and I knew her voice would not get stronger until that part of the cancer had shrunk. However, what did I truly know? I did not ask Joe for more petrifying information. I was afraid he might confirm my worsening fears. Good news was what we all wanted and needed. So I gratefully accepted Joe's reading. I presumed that the brain tumors were the predominant danger and that the cancer would make the journey to healing back along the path from which it came. I asked Joe about that, and he did not discourage me from believing it, but neither did he offer positive feedback.

I wanted to get the comparison pictures of Sybil's lung so we could tell what was happening there. At the same time, I was fearful of the truth. I sent another fax to the Spartanburg hospital requesting Sybil's record. It was our third attempt to get that X-ray. They would not send it this time either. The hospital never responded to any of our requests or inquiries. I was becoming fearful of answers that never came.

The next day, we went to the Tampa clinic. The patients who knew Sybil were anxiously waiting to know the results of her scan. When I wheeled her into the treatment room, she smiled broadly and nodded as I held my hand up in an okay signal. They clapped, and Deedy rushed to greet us with the oxygen tank.

When she and I got Sybil situated, she ordered me, "You come with me. I have some strawberries for Sybil."

As we walked out to the parking lot to her car, she said, "You need to take Sybil to the Strawberry Festival in Plant City, Florida. They have wheelchairs there. I have been using one when I go, because I tire easily."

"Is that where you get the strawberries?"

"Yes," she said and handed me an entire flat of strawberry baskets. "Take these to Sybil. They'll be good for her."

"I'll ask her about the festival. There are too many strawberries here, Deedy," "No, it's not too many. They are good for Sybil. I have some for a couple of other patients who are not eating enough fruits and vegetables."

Deedy was suffering from breast cancer, but that did not keep her from going, doing, thinking, and caring about everyone else. She researched cancer information and shared what she found. She was a bossy woman, but only in the cause of caring for others.

I was putting the strawberries in my car when Deedy told me that Sybil and I should go to a weekly dance in St. Petersburg. "I will ask her about the festival and dance, but I know she will not go."

"She doesn't have to dance. You can just watch and listen to the music. The two of you need to get out and have some fun."

"Thank you so much for the strawberries, Deedy. Thanks for mentioning the entertainment, even though we may not go. It is thoughtful of you to think about our welfare. Sybil does not even want to go out to eat. She's self-conscious about people staring at her because of her condition."

"She doesn't need worry about that. She's beautiful."

"I know, but she's too young to be in a wheelchair. I think that's why she draws attention."

Joan had been waiting at the umbrella table out front. When she saw Richard coming, she rushed to tell him the good news about Sybil's results. I saw his smile when she told him.

When Sybil finished, she was more energetic than usual. While she was in high spirits, we stopped at a bookstore in Tampa, then at Schlotzsky's Deli to pick up lunch to go. We enjoy bookstores, so after lunch back at the camp, Sybil felt up to going to Barnes and Noble in St. Petersburg.

We parked beside the handicap ramp under the shade of a tree, and I performed my ritual of unloading Sybil's chair for her. I was thankful that she had consented to the chair. She could twist her body into the seat with little or no help, yet when she was in the chair and Joan started to push her, Joan realized that Sybil's foot was caught under the footrest. "Oh, my God!" Joan cried out frantically and bent over to remove the trapped foot. I leaned to help her, but Sybil was laughing. She had not felt it.

Joan was upset, so I pushed Sybil into the store. As I wheeled her slowly through the first aisle of books, she suddenly reached out to snatch a hardback book. "For Grandmother's birthday," she said nonchalantly before I could ask. She showed the book to me: *As My World Turns*, an autobiography by one of their favorite soap stars. She and my mother shared their soap opera mania. When they were together, they had animated conversations about the episodes. She tucked the book beside herself in the chair.

She laughed and smiled as we rolled through the aisles. It was pleasant for Sybil, because the clerks and shoppers did not stare. They just greeted her kindly. They were probably more apt to see handicapped shoppers here in a bookstore than in some other places. It was a delight to see her enjoying the excursion. She asked to go to the natural health section where she chose, *Nutritional Healing*. It was a good choice. We would refer to it frequently in the coming days.

Another outing that was not so pleasant was a side trip following our next trip to Tampa. I thought we could treat Joan to a drive and come home a different way. I decided we would take the Courtney Campbell Causeway Bridge to Clearwater and then drive down the waterfront by way of a chain of connecting islands on the Gulf Coast from Clearwater Beach to Indian Shores.

As we crossed over the bridge, Sybil called from the back seat, "I need to go to a bathroom soon."

"I'll stop as soon as I can," I told her.

There was a small welcome center just beyond the bridge. I drove into one of the two vacant parking spaces and hurriedly retrieved the wheelchair from the car's trunk. When I wheeled Sybil up the ramp and into the narrow door, we noticed immediately that there was a long waiting line at the ladies' room. The women stood their ground in line, irrespective of my daughter's obvious handicap. Without a word, I smoothly wheeled her around toward the men's room while the waiting women stared. Sybil looked up at me grinning. It was a private joke between us that Sybil would always choose a vacant men's room when the ladies' room was busy. To her it was a practical choice, and it saved her a lot of misery and aggravation, especially this time. In her present condition, she simply could not wait in a long line of impatient women.

We left to drive across to the Gulf Boulevard, but just as we started toward the small beach towns, Sybil had one of her panic attacks for food. I had not anticipated the out-of-the way trip when I packed her snack pack. She only had a few raisins left.

The journey that I had thought would be a delight along the waterway was taking longer than I expected.

"How much longer?" Sybil asked. I recognized her fear.

"Not long, maybe fifteen minutes," I answered.

"I've got to have something to eat right now. I can't wait!" she cried.

It was the only time Joan saw her in this panicky state. She thought Sybil was having a childish tantrum and said as much. I knew that familiar attack. I never knew why hunger triggered these scary episodes. It was the only time she demonstrated fear. It is strange that it was all about food.

"I'm watching for a store."

I was particularly anxious, but then I spotted a small convenience store and swerved into the lot and came to a screeching halt near the door. I rushed inside, grabbed a banana, a pack of peanuts, and a bottle of juice. My hands were trembling as I paid the indifferent clerk. I knew that Sybil was trembling even more.

"When are we going to get home?" she asked pitifully when I handed the food to her.

"Just a few more minutes," I said. I hoped to calm her, even though I knew it would take us a half hour or more to reach the campground. Fortunately, when she finished her snack, she fell asleep.

Back at the campground, I parked in the shade, rolled down the windows, and left her to rest in the car with the door on her side open. Joan and I sat under the canopy in front of the car where we could see and hear her.

Joan left for North Carolina the next day. Later Joan told me, "When I left Florida, honest to God, she looked so fabulous. She did. She looked so good. Her color was good, her mind was alert, and her sense of humor was still there. I truthfully thought she was getting better. I did."

Sybil and I thought so, too. Unfortunately, Sybil's pain became more severe. Until this time, she had only taken half of a Percocet tablet. Now she needed a whole one. I asked Joe about acupuncture. He approved and recommended Jann, the nurse who worked with him in Tampa.

Jann's practice was in the Vivid Medical Health Clinic in St. Petersburg, located near Joe's treatment center. The surrounding area encompassed a number of medical and alternative medical offices as well as a hospital. She gave us an appointment right away.

I was glad that Sybil was eager to have acupuncture. We were both hopeful. The morning of her first session, she had a severe headache, and we told Jann about that. She helped me boost Sybil from the wheelchair up to the side of the treatment table, where I helped her remove part of her clothing to slip into a backless gown. When Sybil lay down, Jann started deftly inserting the tiny needles. I noticed she placed one in the very top of her head, a tender spot, but Sybil did not flinch. Nor did she move as Jann carefully placed more needles in strategic places, including Sybil's right arm and leg. Then she covered her with a thin white sheet and left the room, putting me on watch to see that Sybil lay still. We joked about her being a porcupine as she relaxed. I was amazed at how quickly she fell asleep. I read a book. Sybil slept until Jann came back and began removing the needles.

"My headache is gone," Sybil announced with delight.

"That's great! You did good, Jann." I was impressed that she had been so gentle while inserting and removing the tiny sharp needles. I forgave her for the earlier incident in Tampa when she did not help Sybil to the bathroom.

We made another appointment with Jann before we left the office. Sybil felt so much better after the therapy that she was anxious to continue. I was happy to have finally found something for her that was truly helpful.

In our next Sunday weekly report, we gave the news of the scan. "3/11/01. This week a CAT scan revealed one small brain tumor on right side is gone! A larger tumor on the left side reduced in size! More to go in lung etc., but Sybil is moving steadily on the Road to Recovery. We thank you with all our hearts for your continued prayers and moral support. Sincerely, Iris and Sybil."

Because we wanted to return to North Carolina, we had been searching for a doctor near home who would consent to administering Albarin to Sybil. While Bill searched at home, I made telephone calls to the area. There are many alternative care clinics in western North Carolina and some in our home county, but we needed one that would agree to administer this particular clinical trial formula. Through some of my inquiries, I had discovered a doctor in Landrum, South Carolina, only thirty miles from home, in the town where our beautician, Gaston Free, has a salon. Sybil and I had made that Landrum trek each month, which always included a stop at Side Street Pizza after a haircut. It would be a good place to take her for further treatment.

I called Mitchell Ghen, DO, of the Biogenesis Medical Center. The center "offers supportive measures for detoxifying the body and to enhance the immune system using a variety of treatments including nutritional supplementation and chelation therapy." I spoke with Dr. Ghen and actually made two separate tentative appointments for Sybil. He was critical of Albarin, but he agreed to see her if she was willing to participate in other alternative treatments. I had hoped he would be familiar with Joe and Dr. Danhof's research. He seemed unaware of the product and the trial.

Bill called one evening to say that he had found a doctor who would continue Sybil's treatments, Robert G. Crummie, MD, a psychiatrist at the Raintree Clinic. The clinic is a private comprehensive mental health center located in Rutherfordton, only five miles from Sybil's home.

Dr. Crummie told Bill that he would come to Sybil's Forest City home to do the procedure. A chill went through my body. I took it to be a good sign and encouraged Bill to accept the doctor's offer. But many times since I have wondered if that chill was a warning I failed to heed. Why did I not think more than one way? I only wanted *hope*.

Bill set in motion plans for Dr. Crummie to administer the intravenous formula to Sybil on her return to North Carolina. Unbeknownst to me, the doctor had told Bill that there was a great possibility that Sybil was going to die. "You just have to be prepared for it," he said. Bill had replied, "Well, you know we've been pretty much prepared for this anyway. Because either you are going to get better or you are not. You're only going to go one of two ways." I never knew how Sybil felt or whether she had discussed this with someone else.

Meanwhile it was still comfortable when Sybil and I were alone. She could communicate with me using only a few words.

I remember an occasion when she had had enough of her snacks. "I'm hungry," she announced one afternoon after her nap. I instinctively opened the refrigerator door and pulled out a plastic container of sliced chicken breast. I handed it to her casually. Suddenly she threw the entire contents on the mobile home floor and declared vehemently, "I'm sick of chicken!"

Frankly, I had not stopped to think of how often I had put the bland white meat in her snack pack. After all, she had morning and afternoon snacks every day between meals. The majority of our meals had been chicken. Though I tried to prepare it in different ways, it still was plain white chicken meat. In some cases it was turkey, which was just as tasteless without condiments. She had been very patient, all things considered.

117

Her outburst was upsetting but she got my attention. Her frustrations were much more serious than a portion of meat, of course, but it helped her to expel some of that anger. She felt better afterward. From that day forward, I purposely tried to avoid any repetition of snack foods, choosing a variety of nuts, fruits, and meats. She and I often laughed about her "sick o' chicken" flare-up in the days that followed. I was glad that she felt free to vent with me.

I continued to shop for medicine and groceries during Sybil's treatment time. And I hurried daily a couple of blocks to the little campground post office to retrieve cards, letters, and packages for Sybil. Family and friends sent books, phone cards, bath and body supplies, gift certificates, and more presents that were thoughtful. All those kind thoughts were very meaningful to both of us. We felt loving fellowship surround us even though we were living alone.

In addition, we had a wonderful surprise visit. Our granddaughter, Hannah Marie, came with her mother, Katherine, and her maternal grandmother. We were so happy to see the baby. Unfortunately, Sybil could not hold her grandchild, but she had the pleasure of watching her. We both thought Hannah looked like her dad, Brian. Hannah was content as long as she saw her mother and had her back to this strange great-grandmother who was holding her. Their pleasant visit was a great treat for Sybil, though she was very tired afterward.

I will always be grateful to Katherine for bringing Hannah to see Sybil. It was such a precious highlight during her confinement. It was the last time she would see her granddaughter.

When Bill told us he was coming back to St. Petersburg, I thought that he and Sybil should have some time alone, so I gave myself a weekend off. I was often too close to tears that I did not want to shed. I felt that a short break from giving care was in order. I needed to renew my spirits for everyone's sake. It would be good for them and me if I excused myself for a couple of nights. Bill and Sybil had not had any private time since she came to Florida.

I drove along the Gulf of Mexico through North Redington

Beach and Madeira Beach on my way to the Holiday Inn on Treasure Island. All the rooms at the hotel have views of the beach and private balconies. My view of the white sandy beach was distant but lovely. I was restless in the quiet room, so I looked in the hotel directory to see if there were any events on the premises. The rooftop restaurant and lounge offered a cocktail hour with wine and hors d'oeuvres. I had enough time to shower and dress.

The buffet of treats on the hors d'oeuvres table was impressive. I was not sure what to choose. I was absorbed in my decision-making when suddenly I realized that I had almost walked into someone who had stopped in front of me. I looked up into the most beautiful blue eyes I have ever seen. He was smiling at me in amusement. The other features of this tall handsome stranger complemented his gorgeous eyes. He spoke, and we were immediately engaged in a friendly conversation, as if we were long-time friends. Then we automatically sat down beside each other at the bar.

"I'm John Gallagher," he introduced himself.

His name was all he needed to tell me. It seemed that I already knew his character and that he was at this particular time and place for a purpose. Moreover, I later recognized that purpose as a part of the respite that I was seeking when I hit the road for the weekend. It worked for me.

John asked, "What brings you to Treasure Island?"

"I'm just over here for the weekend. My daughter is taking treatment for cancer at a clinic in St. Petersburg. When her husband came down to visit today, I took some R & R to give them time alone and to refuel my own energy. And you?"

He told me that they came here every year from Boston. While we were talking, several individuals came by to speak to him.

He asked about Sybil's condition and I found myself pouring out my heartache. I shared my hopes and fears with him. I had not talked with anyone about my fears, but I found that I could talk with this stranger without reservations. Perhaps it was easier because he was a stranger. He also shared a confidence with me regarding a personal family illness.

John was sincerely concerned and promised to pray for us. He wrote his e-mail address on a napkin and asked that I keep in touch about Sybil's condition. John recommended a good restaurant nearby, and then he excused himself and joined a couple across the room. Our conversation provided a respite on my journey through a turbulent sea, a raft tossed gently by a stranger or maybe an angel.

Early the next morning, I called Sybil and Bill. Everything was fine; no need to worry, they said. I left the room to drive to John's Pass village and boardwalk, just south of Madeira Beach. I browsed aimlessly through the shops and then found a tall table at Sculley's Restaurant and watched the water slap lazily against the pilings along the boardwalk. While I mindlessly dined on a plate of calamari and sipped a beer, I thought of the many angels God had sent to Sybil and me. The cast was awesome, and they were from everywhere: North Carolina, Ohio, Iowa, Texas, California, Florida, Virginia, and now Massachusetts. Because of all their support and prayers and her own positive attitude, I was certain that Sybil would survive this dreadful disease. I felt sure of her survival, believing strongly that the power of prayer could prevail against all odds. She was still getting cards, letters, flowers, and gifts, both at the clinic and at the little post office at the campground.

I was not so naïve as to believe the road ahead would be easy for her. It was already very difficult. She was beginning to suffer pain and had no use of her right side. Now her right foot often folded inward suddenly when she walked, and she would cry out in pain. We were pleased that she once again had feeling in her right foot, but she often had no control of the way that foot turned. "No, no!... Stop! Stop!" She would scream and point to her foot when we were trying to help her walk. "It's flopping!" Her foot would be turned so extremely that her ankle touched the floor. Every time it happened, which was all too frequent, I felt panic, fearing that she might break some bones. However, I believed it was a good sign that she had feeling where she had not felt before. We thought that when she felt her foot turn, it might have meant some feeling was returning.

We discussed the brain damage with Dr. Mayer. He told us of a new kind of rehabilitation for stroke victims. It was a rewiring of the brain, so to speak. There was a news release by the American Association For The Advancement of Science, June 2, 2000: "Stroke: *Journal of the American Heart Association,* which shows for the first time that a new type of rehabilitation therapy, employed by researchers at the University of Alabama and the Friedrich Schiller University in Germany, involves immobilizing the good arm of a stroke victim and forced the patient to use their bad arm to perform daily tasks. Patients performed the exercises six hours a day for two weeks. When the course of therapy was complete, a brain scan indicated renewed muscle activity in the paralyzed limb … a finding that seems to vindicate scientists' previous theory that the brain can, in fact, be actively rewired."

"Sybil, sometimes you misfire. Let's try to rewire you."

When Sybil was ready to pick up her bad leg to walk, I asked her to lift it up high and concentrate on putting it down before she put weight on it. "Talk to it in your mind," I told her. "Tell your leg and foot what to do." When she started to lift her leg up, I would remind her, "Lift it up high and think, baby. Lift, think, and set it down easy."

Our strategy was not professional by any means, but when we took the time to practice the idea, it made a difference. Carefully paying attention to the floppy foot seemed to prevent it from floundering so that she could set it down firmly. There was not always enough time for Sybil to concentrate on each step. Nevertheless, since it seemed effective, she did give her attention to the slower process when she remembered and when time allowed.

Even though we were amateur caregivers, Sybil never regretted not going for chemotherapy and radiation. She and I kept alert by constantly thinking of new ideas to make things work *for her.* Our unending research and the processes of trial and error stimulated our daily self-assurance that there were channels leading toward a cure. We always felt supported by the continuing prayers and encouragement from the home front.

It had been a blessing to talk with John at the hotel, because he was not involved with our situation directly. Nevertheless, I was ready to get back to my role as nurse and companion.

Bill had brought his bicycle along with him and was anxiously waiting for me at the motor home so that he could go for a ride in the park. Sybil was in good spirits and listened eagerly to my report of the weekend retreat. She was happy that I had met someone for pleasant conversation.

Bill's trip to the park gave me the idea that we should have a picnic there. The next morning, we drove over to Einstein Bros. Bagels and bought bagels, juice, and coffee for a morning treat in the park. The weather was perfect. A family of ducks entertained us as we sat at a table near the water and ate our breakfast. We sat for a few minutes after the meal, and then Sybil had to go to the bathroom, which was up the hill from us. After the difficult and tiring uphill trek, she was ready to go back to the motor home.

Even though Sybil had been bathing and shampooing herself, I realized that Bill was bathing her now. It took less time and was thoughtful of him to do it. He and I shared the responsibility of tending to her when she cried out for help during the night. He would crawl down from his bunk to help, and occasionally he stayed with her for the rest of the night.

Bill chose to stay in the clinic treatment room during Sybil's therapy and chatted with the other patients. Deedy got his attention when she praised the benefits of juicing fruits and vegetables. By the time the treatment session ended, the idea of the process had hooked Bill. He wanted to go directly from the clinic to buy a juicer.

Our first stop was Service Merchandise. Sybil did not like the price of sixty-nine dollars.

"It's too much," she protested. "We can't afford it."

Bill was attempting to persuade her when I interrupted.

"Sybil, you have a gift certificate for Target that Marce sent you." I suggested that we see if they had one within the price range of the gift card. "The juicer would be a gift from Marce. She'd like that."

"Yeah," she smiled, "she would. If Target has one, we'll get it."

When she agreed, Bill spun her wheelchair around toward the exit of Service Merchandise. "Okay! Let's go to Target."

The Target store was only a mile or two away. Sybil was delighted to find a Juiceman there for a few dollars under the amount of the gift certificate. (*Thank you, Marce.*)

Bill could hardly wait to try out his new toy, but he took us home before he went to the produce stand nearby. He brought home a bounty of fruits and vegetables to test on the new machine and tried them all. The strawberries Deedy brought found their way to the juicer as well, much to my dismay.

It seemed to have happened overnight that Sybil could no longer wear her contact lens. She had some old reading glasses that were a slight help, but she was not able to read as much as she had been. She could still see her daily "dark movies" (that's what Randy called the soaps), and even if she was not watching, she enjoyed listening. She often simply listened to them as she rested in bed.

It was frustrating to Sybil that she could no longer snail mail, email, read books; especially her Bible, where she had marked many passages. She started to sleep longer and more often. We agreed to make an appointment with her optometrist as soon as we went back to North Carolina, which would be soon.

Bill noticed one of the Cushing's syndrome symptoms that I had not noticed. He was watching her apply makeup at the table by a window that reflected light on her face.

"Are the steroids that you take causing you to grow a beard?" he asked.

She glanced in the mirror and brought her left hand up to stroke her face. She and I had not noticed, and I was sorry that Bill had, because on her next trip to the bathroom she got a razor to shave her face. As I watched her cautiously slide the razor across her cheek, I unintentionally shook my head.

Sybil had already reduced her intake of dexamethasone, and now that she was so anxious about the side effects, she wanted to taper off even more.

Dr. Crummie planned a trip to St. Petersburg to learn the treatment procedure from Joe. We were excited about his coming, because it meant we would be going home to continue Sybil's therapy. We truly felt that she was doing well with the aloe regimen and thought that she would improve even more at home. Sybil was also anxious about the rising costs of our extended stay and looked forward to getting some relief from those costs. Many friends and family members had donated money, and we were all grateful for their thoughtfulness.

Once Dr. Crummie decided to give Sybil's injections, he and Bill talked regularly. Even so, we did not know exactly when the doctor would come to observe the procedure at Dr. Joe's clinic. He gave Bill a general idea, but we were surprised to come into the treatment room one morning and see him there.

"Well, there's Bob Crummie," Bill announced, taken aback while recognizing the robust man casually dressed and sporting a wide-brimmed hat. The doctor watched as Joe measured formula in the laboratory section of the room.

"Is that my doctor?" Sybil asked happily.

"Evidently," I said.

Bill left us to go speak to the newcomer while I wheeled Sybil over to a recliner on the end of the center row. She settled into a chair with her pillow and blanket before Joe brought the visitor over to meet us. Dr. Crummie insisted on giving Sybil her treatment for the day. Joe stood by and watched. The doctor had trouble finding her vein on the first try. Joe offered to take over, but Dr. Crummie brushed his offer aside. Sybil quietly watched as he finally inserted the needle properly. Later I asked Joe, "What do you think of Sybil's doctor?"

"He'll do fine," he assured me, with no further comment. I got the same brief answer from Dr. Mayer. It was obvious that they were not overwhelmed with confidence in this new doctor. Some time after the fact, Joe told me that he had not been impressed with the attending doctor, but when he expressed his apprehension to a member of our family, he got the impression that the family knew the doctor and that this was a family decision. Neither Sybil nor I had ever seen the doctor until he showed up at the clinic. However, I did not go into that fact with Joe. He knew that he had not voiced his impression to Sybil and me.

After the day's therapy Sybil, Bill, Dr. Crummie, and I waited in Joe's empty gym while he finished administering treatments to his current patients. He then joined us to give Dr. Crummie the instructions for Sybil's Albarin treatment. Bill and Dr. Crummie chatted easily while Sybil and I sat with our own uneasy thoughts. When Joe joined us, I only vaguely heard him giving the instructions. I did not mentally record the foreign medical lingo. I wished I had a pen and paper to write it down, but I was more concerned with Sybil's present state. It was past time for her post-treatment nap, and she was starting to nod off. She was tired.

When the training session ended, Dr. Crummie told us that he could start Sybil's treatments in North Carolina the following day. He would leave immediately for the ten-hour drive back home.

I thought we needed more time to prepare to leave. "We can finish her treatments here on Thursday," I said, "and that will give us the weekend before the next injection. Let's plan to do her first injection in North Carolina on Monday. Okay? We have to make plans for our transportation and also Jim's motor home."

"Yeah," Bill agreed, "I need to get with Kenny about his plane and Jim about the motor home."

One would think that we were thrilled to leave St. Petersburg. We were not. Our purpose was not yet accomplished, and the clinic had been a protective shield for Sybil. Joe, Jean, Dr. Mayer, and the patients had held her in a cocoon-like atmosphere. Our neighbor in the trailer next door had brought fresh fruit for her from the huge flea market nearby. And the Campbell's motor home had been tailor-made for her ease of movement. Going home would be an uprooting that would require a total readjustment.

Circumstances had changed tremendously during our absence from home. It was necessary for Bill to return ahead of us to arrange for Sybil's return as a patient. The huge spacious house was not handicap friendly The tub and shower combo was an obstacle that Sybil could not conquer alone. Bill would need to acquire a seat for the bathtub, a wheelchair that could pass through the hall to the bedroom, a supply of Depends, a bedpan, a stand for the intravenous fluid container, and a number of household staples. We could not simply walk Sybil through the door without preparation.

Before leaving St. Petersburg, Bill called Kenny, who graciously offered a third round-trip flight. Bill would fly down with a crew to pick up the car and motor home; Sybil and I would be on the return flight with Kenny and George.

Bill suggested we call Randy, who was now working in Spring Creek, Florida, for his friend there, and ask him to come help Sybil and me prepare to leave. When Randy agreed, we were thrilled. He came to the campground a few hours after Bill left for North Carolina. It was wonderful to have him back. We had missed him more than we realized. Sybil was excited that he brought his dog, Fargo.

The three of us went for Sybil's last treatment with Jann. It was sad that those sessions had ended, because Sybil looked so peaceful and relaxed after the acupuncture. Then there was the thirty-ninth treatment with Joe. We bid a sad good-bye to all the friends Sybil had made at the clinic. They were glad for her to be going home for treatment but sorry to see her leave. Deedy brought Sybil two more large boxes of strawberries and a variety of other fruits.

Randy was happy to see their mutual friends at the clinic again and to have another chance to tease Jean. He picked up the vial of Albarin that Joe had ordered for us to take back with us. Dr. Crummie would extract Sybil's formula from the small container. I felt like we needed a bodyguard for that precious cargo.

Randy was a tremendous help. He stayed with Sybil while I took care of terminating Internet and telephone services, canceling the wheelchair rental, paying the final campground bills, and putting in a change of address at the little post office. I waited for the final hour to return the rented wheelchair. Meanwhile, Randy arranged with the airport to have a chair ready for us to use when it was time for our flight.

Randy was up before daylight, as usual, on our final day. While he left to shower in the community bathhouse, I quietly removed the bunk bed and sofa sleeper sheets. Sybil slept until I started cooking breakfast. She was in a somber mood when she awoke. Try as we might, we were not able to arouse in ourselves the enthusiasm we had shared on our arriving flight. We simply went through the motions. Sybil had less mobility now and needed help getting in and out of the shower and the bathroom. She could no longer swing herself by the door into those cubicles. That had happened only recently. Moreover, she had been unable to use a walker for three weeks now. In spite of those changes, we persistently held on to hope.

After breakfast, Sybil lay back on the couch and listened to the television, which now looked blurry to her. I left her with Randy and went once more to the laundry with our bed linens and a few personal items. When I returned, it was a joy to see that Randy and Sybil were joking with each other. It was typical of Sybil not to stay in a down mood for any length of time. She was sad about leaving but glad that she would be seeing her sons and other close family members whom she had missed.

Randy and I checked the camper for items that might become flying objects during the drive back. We expected Bill and Jim to drive the motor home back as fast as they had driven it down originally. Bud was also coming on the trip. One of the three would drive the car back. We tucked the few iffy items safely away and then packed an ice chest with water and sandwiches. I put extra munchies in Sybil's floral snack pack, leaving only enough space to zip it shut.

"Should be enough for the trip," I mused aloud. Sybil nodded with a smile, indicating that she felt secure about it.

As we drove through the Holiday Campground gate for the last time, Sybil waved her left hand gaily, "Good-bye, campground."

It would soon be good-bye campground for the permanent residents there also, for the property was to be sold to a developer and converted to condominiums, causing heartbreak for those who had permanent spaces and for the snowbirds who had wintered there for many years. Thankfully, it had been there for us.

"It was a good place to be," Randy commented.

"Thanks to Jim and Sherry," said Sybil, acknowledging her friends.

Our route to the airport began in the same direction as our Tampa trips, along Park Blvd. toward Gandy Bridge, but then we turned onto Roosevelt Blvd. just before the bridge. When we reached the airport Randy turned off onto a side street and drove to the Signature Flights building, which sat at the end of the neatly landscaped drive. It was an impressive glass front building with stone pillars holding a roof. He then left us in the shaded car while he went inside to get a wheelchair for Sybil. It was a lovely sunny day, perfect for our flight.

"Chad is going to pick us up at the airport," I told Sybil.

"Bless his heart," she said softly.

Chad was like another son to Sybil. In our family album, there is a dear photo of Sybil in her beautiful wedding dress holding a toddler, her nephew Chad, in her arms. Now he worked for Bill in his furniture refinishing business. Since the shop was on their home property, Chad often had lunch with Sybil and her family. She always had a plate for him. She laughed fondly when telling me that Chad would check with both his mother and Sybil to see what was being served for dinner before he decided where he would eat in the evening.

Randy brought the wheelchair out for Sybil. Together we helped her settle into the canvas seat. I rolled her into the building while he drove the car to a parking lot.

The waiting room for private planes away from the main terminal was spacious, bright, and clean. A lovely young dark-haired girl was behind a smooth tall ticket counter on the left side of the room. She was the only one in the room. We had the well-groomed lobby to ourselves.

"Hey," Sybil said, "this is a VIP lounge."

"Of course, that's because we are VIPs."

I pushed Sybil over beside a wingback chair, facing the coffee table that sat in front of a sofa. The landing strip visible through the huge window was a lovely backdrop for the furniture.

When Randy came in, he went around the corner to brew himself a cup of tea, and then he went over to the counter to select a cookie from a basket of sweets sitting there. He leaned against the counter to eat his cookie and started a conversation with the young woman, who responded with a bright smile.

We waited rather impatiently. Sybil and I went down a hall to the restroom. "We'd better go before our chariot arrives," I suggested. I noticed she seemed tired.

I returned her to the lobby and found the tearoom. I brewed two cups of tea and then picked up a couple of sweet rolls from the basket. Randy was still talking to the receptionist.

We had just finished our tea when Randy announced. "Here they come."

"Our angel wings have come for us, baby," I whispered. She smiled weakly.

Helping Hands

We watched the trim Cessna glide easily to a stop. Bill, Jim, Bud, George, and Kenny popped out of the door one by one and rushed toward the building. Despite our reservations about leaving, Sybil and I were excited to see them and welcomed the delightful hugs and greetings. Randy gave solid handshakes and broad smile.

Sybil and I were happy to see our personal "angel wings" again. However, Sybil's frail appearance came as a shock to Kenny and George. But even though the physical deterioration in her was obvious to them, they managed to keep their astonishment in check. She had been on her feet and moved with minimal help when they brought us to St. Petersburg, but now she sat in a wheelchair, nodding slightly and dramatically worse.

Randy pushed Sybil's chair to the waiting plane. It was difficult for George and Kenny to lift her limp body, now dead weight, into the aircraft. She was glad to be flying again and smiled gratefully when we settled in the same seats we had used on our previous flight.

The trip home was not without hope, but it simply was not exciting like our first flight had been. On the other hand, Sybil would be able to get her eyes checked by her personal optometrist and receive her Albarin at home. We would also be near family and friends, though Bill had asked them not to visit just yet. She would not be able to have the same deluge of visitors that overwhelmed her on that weekend break from the hospital. I planned to stay with her during the day and go to my home at night when Bill could be there to nurse her.

We were quieter on this return flight. Her voice was weak, and she slept most of the trip. I focused on thoughts of finding help for her in our home area. The flight was uneventful; there were no bumps, no sunset, but there was beautiful weather, smooth sailing, and a smooth descent.

As the light plane touched the ground, Sybil suddenly spoke excitedly, "Look! There's Chad!"

He was standing at attention just inside the gate beside a wheelchair waiting for us to touch down. His dad, Mike, watched anxiously nearby. As Chad approached, I could see the nervous apprehension on his face. Mike, too, had a furrowed brow. Nevertheless, when the plane came to a complete stop, they came forth with smiles on their faces.

Kenny and George carefully helped Sybil out of the plane and into the wheelchair. As we moved away from the plane with Sybil, Kenny walked swiftly toward a hangar. Mike left us to run after him, reaching for his wallet as he went. Mike tried to pay Kenny for the flights, but Ken shook his head and warded off the offer with upheld hands. I saw Mike insist, but Kenny shook his head vehemently and swiftly walked away into the hangar.

The pilots gave both time and "wings" out of the goodness of their hearts.

Chad pushed Sybil's chair toward the office building and rolled her inside. When we entered, I asked George for directions to the women's restroom. Chad relinquished his hold on the wheelchair to me so that I could roll her to the restroom. A young woman who was propped against a long counter watched us pass by. She seemed to be listening to Mike and George, who were talking quietly when we left the room.

After the bathroom break, I stopped the chair near Chad. Sybil and I joined the ongoing conversation for a short time. But Sybil was tired.

"Let's go home," Sybil said in a whisper.

I nodded to her, "Chad, are you ready to take us home?"

I had not noticed anything amiss, but when we were in my car, Sybil said pathetically. "Did you see the way she looked at me? She didn't speak; she just stared at me. It made me feel awful."

"I didn't notice her staring. Do you know her?"

"Yes, I know her. She's Sally's sister," she said flatly. "I hate it when people look at me that way. It's even worse when I know them and they don't speak."

"Some people are simply just rude," I told her, but silently I felt like the young girl did not recognize Sybil, because the swelling in her face had distorted her features. That incident still brings tears to my eyes. I could not protect her from that pain. It was as hurtful as physical pain for her.

We chatted with Chad during the rest of the seven-mile trip. When we reached the end of Sybil's long driveway, it was apparent that someone was welcoming her home with flowers.

"Oh, look at the flowers! Someone has been busy here," Sybil exclaimed. Her two large concrete planters at the edge of the carport were filled with arrangements of cut flowers.

When we rolled Sybil's chair inside to her sunroom, there was a huge bowl filled with another display of flowers and several wrapped gifts on top of the table. And through the next door on the kitchenette table was another huge floral centerpiece.

"Papaw, Ruby, and Margaret did the decorating," Chad told us, referring to Sybil's dad, stepmother, and aunt.

"Oh, that was thoughtful of them," she sighed appreciatively.

The house seemed even larger now that we were here and I could physically see the difficulty we faced with Sybil's handicap. *Oh, God,* I thought when I walked in the door, *this home is going to be more of a challenge than I imagined.* With a sinking heart, I looked at all the space in the house. Chad rolled her into the small den. She looked around. Even though it was the smallest room in the house, nothing was close enough for her to hold on to in order to move about. She had planned to set things in this room for her treatments with Dr. Crummie, but now she saw that it did not seem practical for a clinical setting and changed her mind. The odds against Sybil having any freedom of movement here seemed impossible, and this made us very uneasy.

I heard the doorbell ring and went toward the side door just as Sybil's dad opened it. We hugged each other in mutual heartbreak for our daughter.

"I know this has been hard on you," he said sympathetically, his voice breaking as he spoke.

I could not answer. We shared the same sorrow.

That moment was a turning point for me. The tough exterior I had unknowingly built for myself crumbled, and I finally knew that all was not well. Our daughter was in grave danger, a fact that we recognized in that moment of shared anguish.

I stepped aside. "Come on in. She's in the den."

He was anxious to see Sybil right away, and she was thrilled to see him. He brought a huge aloe vera plant that he and Ruby had bought for her. I noticed, with relief, that he showed only how pleased he was that she was home again, and not how shocked he was by her changed appearance. I was glad that he could see her after all those weeks she had been away. Though his voice shook slightly, he spoke lightheartedly in his usual banter and joked a bit.

Charles did not stay long, and knowing him as well as I did, I knew he would be crying before he got to his car. Chad left soon thereafter. Sybil's appearance had done nothing to reassure them. Their discomfort set off an alarm of dread that I had been pushing away. It welled up and nearly smothered me before I suppressed it again.

When she and I were alone, Sybil asked, "Will you take me to the bedroom? I want to see if I can go to the bathroom by myself." My heart ached with the impossible challenges we were encountering.

I helped her from the wheelchair to the edge of the bed and

then scooted the chair away and reached for the walker that hospice had lent us. I started to take her right arm.

"No, I want to do it myself," she insisted. She reached for the bars of the walker with her left hand. The pressure tilted the metal legs downward. Without the control of her right hand, she could not level the walker in order to pull herself up from the side of the bed. She shook her head, frustrated. "Aw, S——!" she uttered angrily. Then turned to me defiantly. "Let me try the chair."

I rolled the chair back in front of her, turning the seat slightly sideways to give her room to swing into it. She motioned me away and took hold of the chair arm, causing it to roll away from her just as she tightened her grasp to pull on it. There were four feet between the chair and the wall, with nothing to stop it from rolling beyond her control. I watched helplessly and thought about the motor home, where she had been more independent. This was so hard to watch. I averted my eyes to tighten my eyelids over tears. Nevertheless, Sybil was determined.

"Stand back. Let me do it."

After several more attempts, she accepted the unfortunate fact that she could not manage alone. She shook her head, and she, too, blinked back tears. She held her arms up to me for help. We took the opportunity to give each other an encouraging hug, and I held her tight as I raised her off the bed and into her chair. I realized that the house was not ready for a handicapped person. I wanted to run away with her, to take her back to the cozy, hopeful place we shared in St. Petersburg.

Sybil never relied on someone to do for her what she could do for herself. It was more her habit to take care of others. But now she would have to give up her independence and lean on others for her every need.

I slept with Sybil in her king-size bed that night. I was pleased that she slept well in her own bed and only needed help once during the night to go to the bathroom. Fortunately, she did not need anything for pain that night.

Bill, Jim, and Bud were back early on Saturday with the motor home and Sybil's car. Once his friends left, Bill was free to take Sybil for an eye examination.

When Bill and Sybil came back from Dr. Turner's office, Bill told me that the doctor ordered a pair of inexpensive reading glasses that I could pick up the first of next week. He would wait until later to get prescription glasses. I did not question that decision.

"That's good," I said to Sybil, "you can see your soaps next week."

She seemed unenthusiastic; her mood was depressed. It was obvious that her examination had not been a routine one, but we let it go. When I tried later to get the record of that visit, it was no longer available.

"When can I pick up the glasses, Bill?"

"They'll call when they come in."

There was a lot of catching up to do in both households, though Bill had done well managing their home while we were away.

Since Bill was free to be with Sybil on Saturday afternoon and Sunday, I took her car for a state inspection and then my own vehicle. There were prescription refills to pick up for Sybil and health supplements to get from the health food store. I had a basketful of mail to review, and there was more mail for Sybil, which she would not be able to read without glasses.

One of the biggest obstacles for Sybil was the same as our bathtub ordeal at Grant Motel in Florida. Bill had put a bathing chair in their tub, but it took two of us to bathe her. Bill showered and sponged while I held her. It was hard for her to accept after having had the freedom to bathe alone in the motor home.

In spite of Bill's request for no visitors, quite a few of Sybil's friends came to call that first Sunday. Her son Brian came from Greensboro to be with her. Teresa came with Bud and gave Sybil a manicure. Other close friends popped in as well.

The following week I went to pick up Sybil's glasses at the eyewear store adjoining Dr. Turner's office.

"I want to pick up my daughter's glasses," I told the young girl behind the glassed in counter. "Sybil Yount."

What should have been a simple errand suddenly became a terrible ordeal for me.

"She'll have to come in to have them fitted," she told me.

"She can't come in; she is very sick. I can try them on in her place."

"No, she has to come in herself to fit them."

"I'll try them on. I just told you she can't come here." My voice rose.

She was adamant. "She will have to come in. I can't fit them on you."

That is when I lost it. My wall of resolve crumbled, and I shrieked out in angry frustration. "These are only cheap reading glasses. I told you she couldn't come in!" Now tears were streaming down my cheeks. "My daughter may be dying!" I shocked myself. I had never said that to anyone. I had never before dared to think it. And I did not want to think it now, either. It just welled up from deep inside my being. My grief was not as far beneath the surface as I believed.

The clerk was noticeably impatient with my furious outburst and seemed not to believe me. She retorted brusquely, "Wait here. I'll go get the doctor." I supposed she thought he could reason with me. When she returned alone, I knew that Dr. Turner had simply told her to give me the glasses. She said nothing and simply put the glass case in a bag, printed a bill, then handed both to me. She thought I was being overly dramatic and showed no sign of compassion. In fact, she appeared angry that she had been overruled. I wrote her a check for the total and gave it to her without another word and left.

I got in the car and sat in the driver's seat, sobbing unabashedly, my head bent over the steering wheel.

Sybil put the glasses on, removed them, and never wore them again.

The next day, we were excited when Dr. Crummie showed up to give Sybil the first treatment. He laid out all of his supplies: the needle, white towels, and the vial of formula. There was a stand for the intravenous container beside her chair. It was on loan from hospice. He had no problem inserting the needle this time. As he watched the Albarin flow through the tube, he chatted with us.

I heard David come into the house and went to greet him. I told him that Sybil was getting her therapy, and he chose to go into the den and wait for her to finish. Sybil smiled happily when I told her that David had come. She was anxious to see him.

She was in pain during the treatment. I gave her the Percocet tablet that she asked for. She had only recently begun to take a whole tablet. One pill usually eased her pain for several hours.

Dr. Crummie removed the needle and told us that he would be back the next morning. When he left, Sybil started hurting more and asked for something to relieve the pain. "Honey, it hasn't been that long since I gave you a Percocet. I need to wait a little longer before I give you another."

We waited, but the pain was only getting worse. Soon she was writhing with severe head pain and begging for more medication, something she had never done. I had not seen her in such intense pain. I took her hand, and she squeezed it with bone-crushing strength, begging with her hand as well as her voice. She began to cry out, asking again for something. Helplessly, I tried to talk to her, but she started screaming.

I knew David could hear us. His heart must be breaking for his mother, I thought. He had no way of knowing that this was the first time her pain had been so severe.

I remembered a time at the clinic when she had asked for something between the doses of Percocet. Joe had instructed me to give her an Aleve. I got her one of those caplets, and she smiled gratefully when I handed the tablet to her. Nevertheless, that gratitude was short-lived, for there was no immediate relief. In addition, she was asking for another. Soon, however, she slowly relaxed her grip on my hand and stopped crying out. After a while, she went to sleep.

She was still sleeping when Bill came home late that afternoon.

He and I managed to get her into her wheelchair and roll her into the bedroom, where we put her to bed.

I called Dr. Crummie about the pain and her continuing sleep. He seemed unconcerned. I asked him if he used a stronger formula than what Joe had ordered. "No," he said, "it's the exact amount that Joe told me to use." I doubted him, however, because Sybil had never had such a reaction during or after a treatment.

"She has never suffered like this from any treatment," I told him, "and has never slept this long."

Bill took the phone to talk to him. Dr. Crummie said, "The worst case scenario is that she might die." He told Bill he would come to the house. I felt his response was terribly blunt and insensitive, but I thought that it would be good for him to make a house call. I was wrong.

The doctor went to Sybil's room. When he came back into the kitchen, he nonchalantly sat at one of the barstools beside Bill. I was standing on the other side of the kitchen. He quickly brought up an alarming subject.

"Have you accepted the fact that Sybil may die?" he asked me coolly.

His brusque manner jarred me. I wonder why these doctors want to rip your hopes to shreds and shock your body with abrupt declarations like this. "I … uh … I know that is a possibility," I stammered, trying to shove the notion aside. I stood facing the doctor and Bill, feeling the blood drain from my face as fear spread throughout my body.

The doctor continued. "Bill and Sybil know that she might die. Of course, you know that too. Can you accept that she will probably die?"

I would not acknowledge his suggestion with a reply. I did not want to hear this implication.

Bill laughed nervously and muttered, "Dr. Death." My son-in-law seemed not at all surprised by Bob's cutting remarks. Apparently, they had discussed the dreaded topic before. But Sybil had not mentioned any such discussion to me, and I was not aware of a time when the three of them could have had such a discussion. The fact was that he had not talked with Sybil.

I did not want to hear anymore. The purpose of this meeting was to determine why Sybil's condition had worsened tremendously following Dr. Crummie's treatment. I grew angry and chose to ignore their ominous comments.

"How much of the Albarin did you give Sybil? She has never had so much pain, nor has she slept like this before."

"I gave her exactly what Joe prescribed," he declared.

Bill assured me that he heard the formula during Joe's conversation with Dr. Crummie in Florida and that the doctor had mixed the correct amounts for this first treatment. Now I regretted missing Joe's directions.

Many months later, I had an opportunity to speak with Joe DiStefano in the presence of Dr. Mayer. Joe said, "Sometimes if you give too much of it, you're going to have the pain. It is not going to hurt the patient unless they are frail, then it will. So, even if she had gotten a little more than she should have, it wouldn't have done any real damage unless she got a whole lot more than what she should have. I don't know how much he gave her, but we're talking about tenths, increasing this by tenths, and even if you increase it by one hundredths, which is possible, because it's not too difficult to do that in a little bitty syringe, you have to be careful. So, if he did that, then she would have gotten a little more than she should have. It's not saying that it would have done any real damage, because I don't think it would have, but it would make her very uncomfortable. I don't remember the doctor's name, but he came in and spent some time with us. He seemed to want to believe that he knew a little bit about everything having to do with alternative medicine. I remember him pretty well. He should have known enough to do it properly."

Dr. Mayer interjected, "The thing is, he'd never done it before."

Joe continued. "It's not that difficult to make a small mistake. You have to be really careful in doing the implementations with that solution, and sometimes you actually have to step down the dosage. If you went up and there was a severe reaction, you either stayed at that dosage or you dropped back a quarter of a cc. Now, if you stayed at that dosage and you had the same reaction or greater, then you would have to drop back without question. But if they didn't have a reaction the second time or it was milder, then you could step up the dosage. It was triturated to the patient; there was no real chart saying that this is what you're going to give today, this is what you're going to give tomorrow, this is what you're to give the next day; anything over a tenth of a cc had to be reviewed by the physician in charge; the technicians in Texas were not able to give more than a tenth of cc increase each time, because it was critical to know how the patient would respond."

Dr. Crummie gave us no explanation for what happened with Sybil. His attitude when he left was the same "may live, may die," leaving me feeling worse for having talked with him. I wished I had not.

Later, Bill called Joe, who gave him the name of a supplement for Sybil. I went to my home to start searching for the recommendation by telephone. I knew it was after hours at our local health food store, but I called the owner, Carol Neely, at her home. She was sympathetic but told me they did not have the product at the store. She suggested an Asheville store. There, too, the store had closed for the day.

Meanwhile, Bill called his mother to come over from her home in Vale. He felt more comfortable having her with him.

The following morning, Sybil was lethargic and having pain again.

When Dr. Crummie arrived for the second treatment, she was still in bed and refused to cooperate with him. Because of her bad reaction the day before, I was relieved. I felt that if too much had been given on the previous day, maybe skipping a dose would help relieve her system of an overdose. The doctor left with plans to come again the next day.

Lib stayed with us during the day and was still there in the evening. She was going to stay over again with Bill, so I went home and gave thought to the situation. Lib was genuinely happy to be able to help, not having had that opportunity while we were away. It made me realize that she was not the only person who wanted to be called upon to do something to help Sybil.

I called Bill and suggested that he let some of our family and friends help with our care giving. Lib and I would alternate with other helpers: Sybil's friends Jayne and Sandra, her sisters-in-law, Barbie and Lynn, and my granddaughter, Brooke. Bill readily agreed and immediately set to work on a schedule, then made calls to set it up.

Sybil was happy with the new arrangement. She could visit with people without tiring and sleep when she needed. In addition, it was helpful to me mentally and physically to share the burden of providing care.

It never occurred to any of us to take Sybil to any other place for care. A hospital or nursing facility had all the bells and whistles: a roll-up bed, round-the-clock nursing care, a dietician, and all that stuff designed for the sick. But we never even considered the possibility.

I believed that remedies still mattered, so I shrugged off Bob Crummie's morbid remarks. There was hope as long as she continued on the Albarin and got the proper cancer-fighting foods and supplements. The battle was not over. And I was still searching for other tactics. On the days that I was not scheduled to help, I searched the Internet for some lifesaving miracle. I learned that extracts from mushrooms are in used in Japan for cancer treatment, especially maitake and shiitake. Maitake appeared to be the best.

Maitake D-Fraction and Cancer Growth. Among the various fractions in the process of standardization of the mushroom extraction, it is known that maitake D-fraction is the most potent in enhancing the immune system, thus demonstrating the highest cancer inhibition in oral ad-ministration. Our tests indicate that the D-fraction is very effective in inhibiting tumor growth even at its growing stage. We believe that the tumor inhibition activity of maitake D-fraction is due to its strong ability to strengthen and activate the cellular immune system. It was observed that the production of interleukin-I (which activates T cells) and super-oxide anion (which damages tumor cells) were enhanced. It is confirmed that the cellular immune-competent cells that inhibit tumor growth were strengthened by the maitake D-fraction.

Maitake does not kill cancer cells directly. It stimulates the activities of immune-competent cells and lets them fight cancer cells....

Maitake D-fraction substantially activates cellular immunity, and inhibits tumor growth, prevents tumor metastases (from spreading to other parts of the body), prevents normal cells from carcinogenesis. Some extensive clinical trials using maitake D-fraction and chemotherapy are under way at several cancer treatment hospitals in the U.S. I expect the results will be favorable. Again, maitake extract does not kill cancer cells directly. It activates the immune system, the body's self-healing power. (H. Nanba, "The Healing Properties of Hen of the Woods." *Healthy & Natural Journal* 2 (1): 92–93.)

I tried to find the fresh mushrooms and placed an order for the extract online when I could not find it locally or nearby. The Fresh Market in Hendersonville told me on the phone that they had the mushrooms, but when I made the forty-five minute trip, I found that they only had shiitake mushrooms, not maitake. Sybil would not eat them. They tasted horrible sautéed alone.

While I was online in search of natural pain relievers, I discovered that a mixture of 1/3 part oil of peppermint mixed with 2/3 Everclear (190 proof grain alcohol) is good for headaches. I swabbed her forehead and the back of her head with the solution. It was very soothing. She began to call out to me when the

Percocet was wearing off. "I want peppermint." It was a pleasure to administer the formula.

My sister-in-law, Lucy, told me about Hallelujah Acres, a health ministry devoted to curing and preventing cancer and other diseases by following the Hallelujah diet. The institute is located in nearby Shelby. One morning I drove over to the complex.

There is a large main building visible from Highway 180. The parking lot was filled, and only a few spaces were open in front of the building. I parked and went to the front entrance. I was apprehensive. When I entered, I saw a gift store to my left. Directly in front of me was a hallway that branched both right and left; a long table in the center held an elaborate juicing machine, priced at three hundred dollars. *And Sybil had been concerned about spending sixty-nine dollars*, I thought. Beside the table was a huge stack of fifty-pound bags of carrots. Just beyond that display on the right, the door to an auditorium stood partially open, and the voice of a speaker came through it. I peeked inside to see a congregation of a hundred-plus listeners sitting quietly. Everyone focused on a tall slender man who seemed to be giving a personal testimony. The session hours posted beside the door indicated that this program would soon be over.

I turned to walk further down this hall, seeing a row of closed doors, evidently personal offices. In front of one of the doors was a brown-haired woman who seemed to belong there.

"Excuse me," I said as I approached her, "is there someone here I can talk to about this program?" I went on to explain that I was searching for help for my daughter and told her about Sybil's condition. She said that George Malkmus was the man I needed to speak with, but he would not be in town for another week. She gave me a card and number to call back. "We will have another session next week," she told me, "and there is no charge to attend." I thanked her and made a mental note of the date and time.

George Malkmus was a pastor in the state of New York at the time he was diagnosed with colon cancer. He learned to change his diet and lifestyle, an adjustment that saved his life. After full restoration of his body, he had a new vision to tell the world: if we would only change our lifestyle, the physical problems of cancer, heart attacks, diabetes, arthritis, and most other illnesses would be totally avoidable.

The institute offers positive support, seminars, and a school of natural health (self-study on health and healing, juicing, cleansing therapy, enzyme nutrition, and other topics), as well as a total health spa and retreat.

The Hallelujah Acres course of therapy was promising, but it would take time to produce results, and time was not on our side. *This will be a good program when Sybil improves,* I thought. She was already close to the diet, having eliminated meat, dairy products, sugar, salt, white flour, processed foods, and chemical additives. The Hallelujah diet prescribes a daily ratio of 85 percent raw and 15 percent cooked food, with the cooked usually only consumed at the end of the day. I filed the information on that therapy under "later."

Friends continued to call. Some came by the house, but Sybil was sleeping most of the time following her treatments. Pastor Dave Hobson came by one day while she was asleep, and I was so sorry they missed each other. She loved her pastor, who was both an excellent minister and a special friend. He remembered that visit and spoke to me about it later.

"When she got home from Florida, one day in particular I went over; she had lain down to rest, and you were there. You were busy cleaning the house and fixing ... and the whole family continued with life, the whole family continued with being connected, never once pretending that this was something that you did not need to be serious about. Always very much aware that it was a pinch battle, but never letting it change who you are as far as being family, as being people who loved each other, as being people who appreciated life and who lived each day. I visited with you because I couldn't visit with her; and I went away from that visit thinking, Lord, have mercy, it's more than courage, and there's an inner confidence that's at work here.

"From the time when we got the news from Spartanburg, throughout her treatments in Florida, and through the time she was back at home with the family, it was as if the whole family was saying, probably prompted by her courage, 'Yes, yes, we acknowledge fully that she has cancer. We have no qualms whatsoever about the fact that she's facing a battle that is all uphill, but we're not going to let that stop us from being a family, from loving, from living each moment each day. We're going to deal with that as we live, and we're going to deal with that as we love, but we're not going to stop being who we are because of cancer. It will not change our faith, it will not change our love, and it will not change the presence of God in our lives. It will not diminish our ability to appreciate every moment that we have. Cancer can ravage the body, but it can't touch the soul.' And it had never been more evident with any family."

Sybil maintained her sense of humor in spite of conditions beyond her control that were slowly deteriorating. We found that we now had to use the bedpan when Bill was not at home, because two women could not lift and move her. On one such occasion, she was making unsuccessful swipes toward herself with toilet tissue in hand. Exasperated, she exclaimed, "Somebody moved my butt!" When she found her mark, she laughed about it.

It was a shock when I saw that Sybil could no longer hold her head up on her own. The realization came when she was sitting in a straight chair. Most of the time she was in bed or in the soft lounge chair, where she could lay her head back. I thought it was only occasionally that she had difficulty, maybe when she was exceptionally tired. Other visitors noticed right away.

We discussed another MRI scan with Dr. Crummie. I don't know why I was in favor of it. I dreaded the results, as I had in St. Petersburg. And Bob Crummie's ominous implication had done nothing to boost my positive thinking. Nevertheless, I went along with the decision to have one done. The doctor scheduled a scan for Friday morning, April 13.

Lib, Lynn, and I talked about transportation to the unit at the hospital in Rutherfordton. The girls and I needed Bill's help to lift her, and riding in the car was no longer a good idea for her. Finally, we decided to arrange for an ambulance. Lynn called and arranged for the rescue squad to take her.

My belief in Sybil's recovery changed, even without the MRI results. On Wednesday afternoon, April 11, my granddaughter Brooke and I were sitting with Sybil for her treatment. When Dr. Crummie came in, I introduced him to Brooke, who realized his son was a student in her high school. They chatted about the teachers, school activities, and so on while he laid out his supplies on a white cloth across a small table near the IV stand. He had just put the tie on Sybil's arm and was ready to begin when he suddenly interrupted their conversation.

"I have to go to the drugstore. I'm out of needles."

I was miffed that he was not better prepared. The ordeal was tiresome enough for Sybil without adding additional time to the process. But I said nothing about his negligence.

When the IV process was finished, Brooke left the room for a few minutes while Dr. Crummie cleared away his supplies.

Sybil looked at me, aimed her left hand toward her mouth, but missed it, and whispered, "Numb."

I clutched my heart in fear but said nothing as I noticed the loss of her control of her left hand. I feared there might be a new tumor on her right side or that her last scan had been misread and the original lesion had enlarged. I felt that she might be thinking the same thing. She had experienced the same numb feeling when the other side began. This was a frightening turn of events. Not good. *God,* I prayed silently, *please don't let her lose the use of both sides.*

The doctor did not miss a beat in his cleaning up process and casually gave a medical reason for the numbness that neither Sybil nor I could understand. His nonchalant attitude and calm tone made it sound non-threatening.

He had just let himself out the door when I had a thought.

"Sybil, when Bob realized that he didn't have a needle, he

left the tie on your arm longer than usual. That would interfere with the circulation in that arm and make it feel numb, don't you think?"

"Maybe," she replied softly and seemed to feel better about it. "It isn't numb right now."

"We'll be doing your MRI day after tomorrow, and that should tell us something."

That evening, Lib mentioned the upcoming scan, and I told her, "I don't know if I want to know the results." I was afraid that the smaller tumor might be growing.

"But we'll know what we're dealing with," she replied.

"That's true," I muttered. But now I was truly scared and did not want to know what we were dealing with. In my heart, I knew that the picture would be very bad. I did not want to see it.

Worst Possible Scenario

Most everyone respected Bill's request about visits, included Sybil's brothers, Mike and Randy. Nevertheless I was so frightened by Sybil's pathetic revelation about the numbness on her good side and Dr. Crummie's statement, "Sybil might die," that I called both Mike and Randy and told them to go to see Sybil as soon as they could. I asked them to call their dad with the same message.

I could not sleep that night. If that other smaller tumor was present and growing, she would soon lose use of her other side. It was an unbearable thought.

At 2:30 AM, too late for other phone calls, I e-mailed one of my dearest friends.

"Dear Herb, It rings in my ears like a prediction, 'What is the worst possible scenario?' Your father's crisis advice. I would like not to think of it. However, I think I must. It has not been so good since we are back home. Thank you for your support. I think reality may be worse than I hoped. We will have an MRI Friday morning. Moreover, signs now do not predict as good as I had prayed for … Yet life is hope. Again, my thanks to a special person who I know truly cares for my loved ones and me."

The following morning, I made broccoli soup for Sybil before I went to see her. I was happy to see Mike's car in her driveway when I drove in. He was in the kitchen. We hugged each other.

"I fed Sybil breakfast this morning," he said proudly. Then he smiled as he told me, "She said, 'I'm stubborn. I'm going to make it.'" And Mike believed she would.

"I'm glad you came," I said and put the soup in the refrigerator before going to her room.

She was sleeping peacefully. Without waking her, I leaned over and kissed her lightly on her forehead and whispered, "I love you."

Later that afternoon, Randy came from Boone and stayed with Sybil while Dr. Crummie administered the Albarin. He felt reassured when he left. When I called to ask about his visit, he assured me that she seemed okay.

My golf club, the American Singles Golf Association, was meeting in Asheville that evening. I drove up early so that I could search the area for maitake mushrooms or extract. The Asheville community is a very health conscious community. The mountain climate seems to invite natural healing. Even so, I did not find maitake.

I turned my cell phone off, as is my habit, before I went into the restaurant where my group was gathering. I was free from anxiety for a time during the meeting.

During all my care-giving weeks, I kept my cell phone turned on constantly. No one called as I drove home from Asheville, and I felt reassured that all was well with Sybil. She was safe, because Lib would be staying overnight.

As I walked into my house, I heard the telephone ring and ran to answer.

"Mom!" It was my son Mike. His voice sounded an ominous alarm. "Did you get my message?" I looked at my cell phone, dismayed to find that I had failed to turn it back on after the meeting. I clicked it on and put it in my pocket.

"No, I did not get a message. What's wrong?"

"Bill called, and he took Sybil to the hospital. He said she stopped breathing."

"My gosh!" I cried. "Stopped breathing? She's at the hospital now?" My mind raced wildly. I was suddenly physically ill. I couldn't grasp the horror.

"Yes, Bill is with her. I'm at the lake, and I'm leaving right now to go there."

"I'll be there. I'll leave right now," I said. I couldn't imagine what had happened to Sybil.

According to Lib, Sybil had a good day. She had eaten the broccoli soup for lunch but only a bite or two at supper. Then she was sleeping a long time, so Bill and Lib checked on her every five to ten minutes. Bill called Lib into the bedroom because Sybil did not seem to be breathing, but her heart was strong. Her eyes were closed. There was no sign of pain and no movement. Bill tried to breathe air into her lungs. He called Dr. Crummie, and then he called Joe in Florida, who told him to call 911. Two ambulances arrived promptly from Emergency Medical Service, which was only a mile away. The medics rushed in and worked with her for at least twenty minutes before taking her to the hospital. Bill and Lib followed. "I thought I was prepared for this," he had told his mother, "but I'm not." He started calling family.

Numbly, I put the phone on the hook and went straight to the door. *Mike said she stopped breathing. He did not say whether she started breathing again. Surely she did.* I was detached and drove by instinct. Midway to the county hospital, a ring startled me. I realized it was my cell phone and flipped it open.

"Iris, where are you?" asked Bill.

"I just passed Public Service Company and Haynes Plant," I replied.

"Well, there's no need to hurry. Sybil just died," he announced flatly. "Take your time and be careful."

I did not reduce my speed. I did not believe him. He spoke too matter-of-factly for something so dreadfully critical. I did not stop to wonder why he would tell me that if it were not true. I simply did not think my daughter could be dead; therefore, I would not let it sink in.

I continued numbly toward my goal. All I could comprehend was that my daughter was in trouble and I needed to be with her as soon as possible. That is all I allowed myself to think.

I finished the trip detached from the facts. I had learned how to disassociate, how to refuse to absorb the pain of full realization all at once. I had been there before. I would let the whole story in gradually so it would not hit me full force. It was a way I used to cope with horrendous shock. And so I refused to let all the actuality of this tragedy touch me right now.

After making a mental note of my parking place, I rushed up the hill toward the hospital's emergency room. The receptionist in the lobby sensed who I was and pointed me to a room off to the right where I would find family members. I opened the door apprehensively and took in the occupants swiftly without looking directly at anyone. Chad was with his girlfriend, seated beside Bill. Charles and his wife, Ruby, stood in the center of the room. A nurse sat in a chair facing them. Charles came forward tearfully and hugged me. Then the shock spread throughout my body. I knew suddenly it was true. We were losing our child.

The nurse stepped forward; I now recognized her as Nikki, the daughter of Sybil's friend Teresa. She stood up to put her arms around me and asked, "Would you like to see Sybil?"

Speechless, I nodded yes and followed her out of the room. We passed the nurse's station, and then Nikki led me into a small room. Sybil lay on a high narrow bed with only a sheet over her up to her shoulders. I walked past Pastor Dave and Lib, who were standing beside the bed. When I looked down at Sybil, it was as if I was not there, as if it were a drama and I was in the act. Her upper torso was darkly splotched as if bruised. She was not moving, not breathing, and not in pain, yet the heart monitor was still active and lively. It spiked when I spoke to her. *She is not dead! She waited for me,* I thought, *to say good-bye. Thank you for waiting, Sybil, so that I can tell you one more time I love you.*

"It's okay, baby," I said aloud as I brushed her forehead. "I know you're tired. You can rest now." I continued to stroke her forehead.

A doctor came in and gave the minister a questioning look. Pastor Dave looked at the heart monitor and said, nodding toward me, "It was going down until she came in."

I sensed another presence and saw that it was Chad.

Sybil looked so peaceful, resting quietly without the pain that had become so relentless the past few days. In spite of her anguish, her mind had remained alert throughout her illness, including this morning with Michael. However, there had been the thought in my mind that the sudden lack of sensation she had felt on her good left side two days earlier boded further deterioration of both body and mind. Eventually the tumors, which seemed to me to be growing again, would rob her of all her physical ability. And in time, those lesions would attack her brilliant mind. Sybil would not have wished for that kind of ending to the pleasant life she had led. She would have begged not to be caught in such an agonizing demise. She chose an alternate treatment for that very reason, to avoid the terrible consequences of chemotherapy and radiation. Now she would choose to go before the ravages of cancer could further invade and destroy her dignity. How could I not let her go now to a place without physical limitation, a place beyond the pain and fear? She had waited for me to say good-bye.

Again, I gave her permission to go. "You have been so tired. You can rest now." I bent to kiss her on the forehead.

The pastor later said to me, "Noticing that her heartbeat increased when you came into the room didn't surprise me. She was finishing with this life. She was finishing with this life and beginning another. Her life continued right up to the very moment that her soul found its way home. Her heart continued to beat as her soul found its way home. She was waiting, I think, for you. She wanted everybody to have as much time as they needed to get ready for what had to be."

The doctor was waiting nearby to pronounce her death. My appearance delayed that long enough for me to say good-bye to my child. Then the monitor began to decrease and the line began to straighten. I did not want to hear the final words that the doctor would record, but neither could I leave until he did. I waited until it was over.

It still seemed like someone else's drama as I left the room in a daze to join the rest of the family. Chad and his fiancée were trying, by phone, to find Brian, whose work with UPS required some night work. Bill had contacted David via his cell phone and notified other family members, but he had not yet located Brian.

Oh, no, no, no, my heart cried. Oh, God, my child is gone. No. I do not want this. It cannot be true. It will never be real. Not Sybil, who is always so cheerful, healthy, and lively. Please, God, lead me through this catastrophe.

There was nothing more to do. We had to leave believing that Sybil was gone. When I walked out the hospital door, I saw Mike's car speeding up the emergency drive toward us. I rushed to meet him. He saw me shake my head and knew.

He screamed, "Oh, no!" I put my arms around him, and we held each other as he cried.

He was still trembling when I whispered, "Go see your dad." Charles was waiting on the sidewalk, watching and hurting.

Pastor Dave came out and walked with me to the parking lot. "You strike me as one who does not ask for help," he said, "but if there is anything that I can do for you, please call me." Normally he would have been right, but his offer made me realize that now there was something I could not do.

"As a matter of fact," I replied, "I think I need you to help me right now." I reached for my cell phone. "Will you call my brother, Martin, so that he can call my other brothers and my mother?"

"I'll be glad to," he said and took the telephone in his hand. He waited patiently while I fumbled through my purse for the number. I could not tell anyone aloud that she was gone. Thankfully, Pastor Dave was kind enough to take care of that for me.

Fortunately, Bill had made the calls to his family, though he was terribly frustrated because he had not found Brian.

After thanking Pastor Dave, I drove to the forlorn house where the family was gathering. Even at that late hour, people were coming to Sybil's home. I poured a glass of wine and just stood by, listening silently to the guests. I was in a deep stupor. I felt I was observing a nightmare.

My brother, Harold, and his wife, Lucy, came from Shelby, despite the late hour. Randy was there. The word had passed swiftly, and people kept coming. But not Brian.

Bill was pacing with a telephone, re-dialing impatiently. Finally, he shouted loudly, "Where in the hell have you been? Your mother just died!"

The room fell silent, shocked. Lib broke the silence. "There is really no easy way to tell him." She was right. There was no way to soften the jolt; one quick jab might even be better than trying to lessen the blow. Any manner of learning about such a tragedy is going to wound the heart.

On Friday morning, we found ourselves planning a funeral service, something one never expects to do for a child. Bill, Charles, Shane Early, the funeral director, Pastor Dave, and I gathered in the room where Sybil had taken her treatments to make those untimely decisions. Sunday was suggested as the day for the ceremony, but Bill stated right away, "I don't want to bury Sybil on Easter." It would have to be Monday, the sixteenth. Frankly, I did not want to be dreading the event for that long, but I kept silent. My only personal request was one that had been Sybil's own.

"Sybil did not want an open casket," I told them. "Sybil always said that she did not want an open casket. No public viewing." That was acceptable to everyone. Shane arranged for a private viewing just for the family.

I knew that Pastor Dave and Shane Early would conduct the formal funeral ceremony with the utmost respect for Sybil. I trusted both of the men implicitly.

Bill made a decision about family visitation that would have made Sybil happy. We would see friends at their home on Sunday afternoon. Sybil had never been comfortable with the formality of the funeral home setting for visitations. She and I usually went together to visit bereaved families, and we went as early as possible to avoid long lines. She would like the informality of greeting guests in the home where she had so often greeted them herself.

Shane asked Bill and me to select a dress for Sybil. We both forgot about it until a messenger from the funeral home came to pick up the outfit. We rushed to the bedroom closet and quickly sifted through the clothing there. Each dress I took off the rod for Bill to approve was "too small," he would say. One he said was too tight even before her sickness caused the bloating that left her so much larger than her normal self. I was not pleased with our final choice, but her size was the decision-maker. There was not time to buy her another. I wish I had had the sense of mind to buy her something special. As it turned out, the dress did not matter. At the family viewing, her beautiful waxen body did not resemble her former healthy self at all. The person resting on the puckered white satin cushion was not my precious child. Her lovely spirit was in another place.

Easter Sunday was a beautiful sunny day. A procession of cars began driving in and out of the long driveway that led to Sybil's home. The spacious lawn filled with parked cars. Among the guests were childhood neighbor and friend, Lynn, now living in Colorado, high school friends, college roommates and fraternity sisters from as far away as Texas, and family from all over the state. There were recent acquaintances with whom Sybil had formed an instant rapport, fans and baseball players who were friends of her sons and who for years had cheered with and been cheered on by her as she religiously followed all of the games.

It was late in the evening when the multitudes stopped coming. Sybil's fraternity sisters stayed to visit, sharing memories of her amid laughter and tears. She surely was with us remembering how much she loved those joyous times with her friends. They spoke of her naiveté on her arrival at Lenoir Rhyne College. They were astounded and amused by her innocence and delighted by her positive attitude. Sybil was a loyal, devoted friend and had stayed in touch with them throughout the years, including her recent e-mail communications. After the girls left us, they continued sharing their memories at the local motel until the early morning hours. They sat together at the church the following day.

The funeral. I cannot possibly go to a final service and burial for my daughter. "Dear God, how can I do this?" I cried out in prayer, "Please, please help me get through this day. I know I have to go. I so do not want to."

When Shane drove my mother and me to the front of the First United Methodist Church in Forest City, I wondered if something other than Sybil's funeral was happening nearby. The three parking lots were full, and cars lined the streets in front of, beside, and behind the church. Inside, mourners were standing at the back of the church, and the pews were completely filled.

The processional hymn was one of my favorites, "Amazing Grace," but it brings tears to my eyes. I always remember my late father singing it. Today it was even more mournful as I walked down the aisle with my widowed mother and my sons behind us.

Pastor Dave began speaking from the pulpit: "We have gathered here to praise God and to witness to the faith of the church and to celebrate Sybil's life."

God began to answer my prayer with words from her dear friends. The celebration began with Tommy Hicks's tribute to Sybil. A hush settled over the congregation as our friend, Kenny Hankinson, pushed Tommy's wheelchair down to the front of the church and adjusted the microphone for him to speak.

"Be nice if the preachers would leave for a few minutes while we do this, and everyone under fourteen also," he said smiling. A sound of refreshing laughter rang through the church. "Just kidding. Well, this is going to be the PG version, Charles, Iris, and family. I would like to say 'How're we going to go forward without Sybil?' But if Sybil was here and I said to her, 'How're we going to go forward without you?' could you imagine what she would say? Oh, Lordy, I'd rather go forward than put up with the lecture I would get."

Laughter again rang out.

"Twenty-five years ago," he continued, "I was down and out, clinically depressed, with no hope, fearful of a future filled with obstacles too great to face. My friend Sybil brought me a tiny book entitled *The Greatest Miracle in the World*. I didn't want to lift my head off the pillow, much less read a book. But when one of the prettiest girls you ever saw asks you to do something, you find a way. The book hit a nerve. The greatest miracle in the world was simply pulling yourself up by the bootstraps, putting self-pity in the garbage can, and getting on with the program. I thought she had a lot of courage to bring that book to me, to think that I had a life worth living. She wanted to spread some hope where there was none. My entire life I've credited Sybil with getting me to take that first step to recovery. And twenty-five years later, I can say it's been an interesting, fulfilling, and fascinating run."

He recalled other times that Sybil supported him and other special times they shared.

Pastor Pat Jobe followed Tommy's remarks with a letter from their former classmate, Dr. Tim Luckadoo, vice chancellor of North Carolina State University. "She was a special, one of a kind, stubborn, hardheaded, loving person. Sybil brought spirit to the Class of '72, and her spirit has made us all better people. It has also made us aware of how important our relationships have been and will continue to be. We owe it to Sybil to remain close over the years."

Pat read a tribute from Mike, her twin brother, whose message was about Sybil's optimistic nature. "She always saw the glass half full and not half empty. My exact last words to Sybil as well as hers to me were, 'I love you,' followed by a kiss."

Then Pat said, "Now this next one here is from me. Sybil Yount, when she was Sybil Sechriest, taught me a lot about rejection." The assembly laughed. "Actually," he continued, "Sybil and Toni Shell taught me a lot about rejection." Laughter again. "Well, really it was Sybil and Toni and Debra Gibson and Bobbie Jean Kennedy, Jody Key, Karen Spratt, Vivian Lowery, Becky Hunt, Lynn Whisnant, Rhonda Ingle, Michelle Pearson and Tanya Bruce and Debbie Whittaker and Sherry Allen who taught me most about rejection." There was more and louder laughter. "And Sylvia Vickery and Nancy and Sharon Logan and June Biggerstaff and Debbie Lavender. But it was Sybil who clobbered me in the eighth grade, and, as bad as I hurt then, I have thoroughly enjoyed telling the story. And Sybil was always kind to let me tell it many times in the thirty-three years that have passed." He then told the story about Sybil's friends trying to match him and Sybil when she said "No way."

"I wandered down the hall to see how things were going," Pat said. "This turned out to be a bad move on my part. What I saw from about thirty or forty feet away was Sybil looking my way as the other girls were pointing at me, and Sybil was gesturing wildly with total disgust. No matter how many times I told the story in the years that followed, she was always kind enough to laugh politely and change the subject. Sybil was always beyond kind enough. She lived out a kindness and consideration and gentleness and compassion that are the very essence of what it means to be a follower of Jesus."

A former co-worker, Wavolyn Norville, spoke of her friendship with Sybil: "When she would come in every day, it was like the sun came in with her, and the sun never went down until we left together at five o'clock."

Jayne was trembling when she went to the podium to speak. "See, Sybil, I got up here without tripping. I've got a thousand stories to tell about Sybil, but we won't be here until three or four in the afternoon, and most of them shouldn't be told in church anyway."

The ready laughter in the congregation made it a joy to celebrate Sybil's life, because she would have been so glad to know that we could laugh, and she certainly would have laughed along side of us.

Jayne could hardly contain the tears when she said, "Sybil is my best friend."

She paused, took a deep breath and continued. "From the moment when I went to Lenoir Rhyne and asked the girl sitting by the tree, 'Is this Fritz Dorm?' and Sybil answered, 'Sure is,' we became a part of each other's lives. She was always there for friends and family, No matter what time of day or night, good news or bad; and I tested that one on several occasions. One weekend when she and I had just finished making the barbecue sauce that we made every year, I got a call from my sister-in-law telling me that my mother was very ill and that I needed to go to Maryland. I was afraid my old Volvo wouldn't make it, so Sybil said to take her car. I did, and I was gone a week. It didn't matter to her. Anything she could give you she would."

Bobbie Jean Burrow wrote a poem for Sybil, "True Friends." She and Sybil were true friends throughout high school and still were. They were always as close as the telephone. and spoke often about their classmates, their children, and their private feelings.

Those special tributes to my daughter made her memorial service not only bearable but enjoyable as well. Who would have thought it could be so? I am so grateful for the memories they shared with us that day and for helping us remember Sybil with fondness and laughter instead of tears.

Pastor Dave summed it up: "Those words gave much light and joy and color and dimension to this service of worship of God. It was as if we stood at heaven's gate and walked as far as we could walk with her.

And against our will, we let Sybil go to another place.

The Best Way
A gentle and loving trail

The oncologist had directed Sybil toward two dead ends: the one with no treatment and the other using the toxic chemotherapy and radiation. Both of his directions led to certain death. The third way, the way that Sybil chose for herself, also led to death, but the path was a gentle and loving trail. Of her three options, it was the best way.

It would have been impossible for Sybil to enjoy the quality of life she had in the end had she been exposed to chemotherapy, the invasive and toxic treatment that makes a person worse each day than they were the day before. Her last weeks were painful, but she never suffered the side effects of chemo, such as nausea, diarrhea, and loss of hair, loss of appetite, malnutrition, internal bleeding, and more.

I revisited the St. Petersburg area and was fortunate to be able to talk with Joe DiStefano, Dr. Mayer, and Jean.

Jean remembered Sybil's joy at the clinic.

"She was happy to be there, and it was not just a happy face she put on. You could see a bit of progression when she was feeling better. Any little progress she made, or if she felt better, you could just look at her and see it. I hated to see her go home, really. But she needed to. If somebody was down, all they needed to do was to look at her, and it just brought out the best in people. She certainly did her job there. She was very much missed. I'll never forget her."

Beyond the healing properties of the Albarin was the gift of compassion and faith Sybil received from two courageous men, Joe DiStefano and Dr. Daniel Mayer, a gift which they generously distributed to all who came through their doors. They turned no one away, no matter what their oncology diagnosis.

They talked to me about Sybil.

Joe said, "She had a brain tumor. And, you know, it's interesting about the product. It worked well for most forms of cancer, but brain tumors were where it really didn't work well. But we had about three cases of brain tumors, and the first two did very well. The tumor began to shrink and never got any worse, and I think one of the fellows is still alive. I haven't heard from his brother recently, but every once and a while I'd see his brother and he would stop by and say, 'Hey, my brother's still doing great, and the tumor hasn't gotten any bigger. It's still there; it just hasn't gotten any bigger.' So, you know, if you don't follow through with the study to know exactly how it's going to affect an individual, you don't know whether it's going to work or if it's not going to work.

"But I know the people who came to us with the brain tumors were saying, 'Look, we have no other place to go.' They're telling me 'I'm going to die no matter what, and this seems to be natural. Please let me try it.' So we said, 'Fine, we don't want to turn you away, and it's not going to cost you an arm and a leg. Consequently, we'll let you have it.' You know, at some of the cancer centers up here, it costs hundreds of thousands dollars, and it still doesn't work, and they're getting worse."

Dr. Mayer said, "We didn't have really good results with brain cancer because it seemed that the medication could not get across what we call the blood brain barrier. That's probably why it didn't work as well for Sybil as we'd hoped it might. However, we're of a philosophy here that anything we can do to give people hope is good. Even though we may not know all the answers, by giving hope we feel like this raised the spirits, which is also important. Blood brain barrier is a common medical expression; any medication that you give has to get into the brain cells by passing through what is called a blood barrier. You might think of it as a covering of semi-permeable material that the medicine has to get through if it's going to do any good in the brain cells. But in certain types of cancer, the medicine cannot penetrate the barrier."

"You didn't have good results with Sybil's brain tumor," I said, "but you had excellent results in helping her and her fellow patients maintain their dignity and quality of life throughout their treatment process. Many patients lived, and that made the trial worthwhile, even though it was cut short."

Joe replied, "You know, most of the patients that came here had that. In fact, one of the fellows, he was considered terminal. He had just started the program. They had to wheel him in a wheelchair. He wasn't able to hold his head up, and he couldn't read a newspaper. He loved to read the newspaper every morning, and he wasn't able to do that. He had about six treatments, and from that time on, he was able to sit up and read the newspaper, and he was out of pain; the pain medications they were giving him no longer worked when he came. So we could see where the quality of life came back with the product. Even though it may not have done everything that we would have liked it to do, it certainly did relieve pain and give certain people back the quality of life, and that's one of the rewarding things about it. So we had a lot of good attributes."

At the time I talked with my medical friends in Florida, they were no longer allowed to administer Albarin. The FDA had stopped them just six months after Sybil left the clinic.

Joe's total treatment cost ranged from zero dollars to $1,375. The cost of chemotherapy, by contrast, is enormous. It comes down to a conflict between corporate wealth and public health, as John. J. Moelart puts it in "Cashing In on Cancer":

> No matter how many people shave their heads or run for the cure or cycle all over the place, cancer will contin-

ue to spread in our midst and claim more and more lives so long as prevention is ignored and non-conventional treatment and research are stifled, while carcinogens are allowed to enter into our food, water, and soil. What we witness here is a conflict between corporate wealth and public health. Try to imagine what would happen if an inexpensive cancer cure were allowed to enter the medical market. Such a development would have devastating economic consequences for cancer profiteers who—like TV evangelists—very effectively and manipulatively use hope and fear to raise money. They have fooled the public into believing a cancer cure is just around the corner and all that is needed is money. It is an empty promise, but a great fundraising tool. Millions of people keep donating to the cancer establishment without having a clue what exactly happens to the money. Public ignorance about the politics of cancer is the result of widespread distortion and suppression of relevant facts by the cancer industry, government and mainstream new media. The so-called war against cancer is mostly a hoax. (http://members.Shaw.ca/eye-openers/cashcancer.htm)

And the drug companies that supply the toxic chemotherapy, I might add, are also to blame.

Deedy wrote to me to tell me that Joe's clinic was raided by the FDA and that she and other patients from the clinic were protesting at the courthouse in down town Tampa. The rally was covered by Josh Zimmer of the *St. Petersburg Times*:

Patients Rally for Alternate Therapy

Patients of Joseph DiStefano are angry over the shutdown of his alternative medical treatments. They are trying to raise money for an attorney and will take their case to Congress.

CARROLLWOOD—They gathered near a courthouse in downtown Tampa, carrying angry signs about the government, wearing pins that said "Ain't Dead Yet!" and worrying about survival without their alternative medical treatments. Patients receiving aloe vera-based cancer treatments said their lives were thrown into disarray Oct. 11 when federal agents raided alternative clinics in Carrollwood and St. Petersburg.

Armed with search warrants, authorities seized serum supplies and patient files from the Medical Center for Preventive and Nutritional Medicine in Carrollwood and St. Petersburg. Agents also took materials from practitioner Joseph DiStefano's house in Largo, effectively stopping a treatment he and others credit with improving the health of cancer patients and perhaps curing some.

Agents came from the U.S. Department of Health and Human Services, Florida Department of Law Enforcement and the Hillsborough County Sheriff's Office. U.S. Attorney's Office spokesman Steve Cole would not comment on the investigation. U.S. Judge Thomas McCoun III sealed the search warrant affidavits, which contain the evidence used to justify the search warrants, for 120 days. (October 26, 2001)

John C. Hammell, president of International Advocates for Health, wrote of the incident in *Life Extension* (April 2002).

In this article, we report on recent FDA raids against alternative clinics that offered a treatment that appears to be effective. The harsh reality is that because the FDA summarily banned this treatment, cancer patients who were using it may now needlessly die.

One of the reasons you read *Life Extension* magazine is to learn of facts not reported by the mass media. The news you haven't heard about is that the FDA continues to attack those involved in innovative medicine, despite the documented failure of mainstream oncologists to save the lives of their cancer patients.

Unlike charlatans who sell worthless products to terminal cancer victims, nutritionist Joe DiStefano, Daniel Mayer, DO and Ivan Danhof, MD, PhD, seemed to be doing everything right. They had discovered a non-toxic therapy that appeared to be prolonging survival time.

Joe DiStefano, Drs. Mayer and Danhof were attempting to file the cumbersome paperwork with the FDA in order to conduct a formal clinical study. They did not advertise or promote their product, nor did they promise any miracles....

Cancer patients given a death sentence by their oncologists appeared to be getting better when using this natural therapy. There is also evidence in the published scientific literature indicating that this therapy might be effective. Based purely on word-of-mouth, a growing number of terminal cancer patients began to seek out this low-cost, and non-toxic, and possibly effective natural therapy.

According to the FDA, none of the above was permissible. The FDA has taken particularly brutal steps to make sure that no cancer patient can access this therapy. The FDA wants to criminally indict those involved so that this therapy will never be available.

Three years after the ordeal, it was still fresh and distressing for Jean. "They came and they said, 'Anyone who would like to be released from this treatment, we're here to take care of you.' They brought in from the county a six-ambulance crew in there with stretchers, defibrillators, IVs, and such. They said, 'You don't have to stay here and have this stuff.' Somebody said, 'We don't need you guys. Jean's here.' 'We're here to take the IV off,' they said, 'We don't want the IV off.' So they had to wait. They couldn't do anything. They made Dr. Mayer go outside in the hot sun. They pulled all the phones, took all the charts, and they took the stuff," Jean said sadly.

Paul Schebell, who had been seeing marked improvement during his treatment, said, "Why don't you get out of here and leave us alone?"

"This will be your last treatment," the agent emphatically stated. Paul slumped in his chair, but when Jean tried to go across the room to comfort him, the FDA agent blocked her path. She pushed past him and went over to Paul.

They need not have treated them like criminals. Two men would have sufficed to deal in a civilized manner with Joe and Dr. Mayer, who would have conformed to the law. They need not have involved the patients, who were there as a last hope for life.

"The patients were horrified," Jean said. "Paul's mother started crying and said, 'Please don't take this away from him.' He just looked at her and said, 'Sorry, I have to do my job.' And Paul just cried. I felt so bad for him."

Hammell related the events that took place in the weeks before the raid:

In early October 2001, Joe DiStefano exited his clinic at midnight after a long day's work, and was startled to hear strange noises coming from the dumpster in the back. Trash was strewn all over the ground. He peered over the top of the dumpster and caught two strangers red handed, with rubber gloves on, probing through his dumpster....

When Joe demanded to know who they were ... they would not identify themselves and had the nerve to say "we're looking for boxes." "Sure you are," said Joe, "everyone looks for boxes at midnight in a dumpster with rubber gloves on." Joe proceeded to write down their license number in order file a complaint with the St. Petersburg police. He demanded that they put the trash back, which they did only grudgingly.

The next week, 120 agents raided Joe's clinics in St. Petersburg and Tampa and his home. Joe's personal property, including his children's computers, was seized while the agents made insulting comments to Joe and Georgiana. At the same time agents were raiding Joe's home and clinic, raids were conducted against Ivan Danhof in Texas and the pharmacist who prepared the aloe extract, Jerry W. Jackson of Allied Pharmacy Services.

Joe is still hurt and saddened by the invasion that terminated his clinical trial of Albarin. He talked to me about it as Dr. Mayer sat with us.

"We've just seen some remarkable things here," Joe said. "It's just sad that we can't do more. But I do understand that Dr. Danhof is still studying it and is in the process of trying to get it approved in Texas. They won't allow it to be shipped across the state line anymore. Therefore, we are unable to help people with it. And it was help in the time we were here. We've seen remarkable things.

"One girl had a tumor the size of a grapefruit in her liver, and I mean she spent hundreds of thousands of dollars for procedures, and it was just getting bigger and bigger, and she started here, and it began to shrink and it went to nothing. Remember that case?" Joe turned to the doctor.

"Yes, I do," Dr. Mayer replied, nodding.

"I can't mention the names because of the privacy act, but we've just seen some remarkable things here. We were seeing tumors shrink, prostates shrink, and so on. And as time went on, these people were, of course, going back to their oncologists telling them they were coming off their medications. Their tumors were shrinking, and they were getting back to normal.

"And it seems as though someone took exception to this fact and filed some complaints with the Federal Drug Administration. That's when they decided that they were going to come in here, and rather than asking questions the way they would normally do, they came in here with swat teams and confiscated everything we had and stopped me from using the drugs totally. Since that time, some of the individuals who started the program late of course passed away because they no longer had the product. But those who had been on the product for a couple of years are still alive and doing well and have beaten their cancer.

"We have two of them coming in routinely. Two of them were in here just a couple of days ago, and their cancer has never returned, so we know that it had a tremendous impact on cancer. We were never able to put together all the data and information, because it has been confiscated."

"And so they have Sybil's records also?" I asked.

"Absolutely. They belong to the clinic or the patient. The patient actually owns their own records; the clinic is the custodian of the records, and they came in with a search warrant and took everything."

"So there's no way for even the patient's family to get those records?"

"Not unless they petition the government, the federal government. The federal government will make you copies of it. You won't get the original records. As of this date, nothing was done, and they haven't pursued it, so that's been over two years now. It's just hard to say; the federal government doesn't want to return anything to us. We can't get our supplies back. We can't get anything back, so we just don't know what that situation is going to entail.

"We had a drug company come in who wanted to purchase the rights to it. They sent a team in here. And there were five or six people. They spent weeks with us talking to patients and watching the procedure etc., and they were so enthused. They could not believe what they were seeing and what they were hearing from the patients. And they wanted to use the product in conjunction with another product that they were marketing for cancers. They felt that putting them together would work out well. They had some original contact with Dr. Danhof and were getting ready to make some sort of offer, but in the interim the government came in and stopped everything, and they backed away from it. So there was interest. They would have never continued with their interest if they had not come in here and seen firsthand what was going on.

"We were dedicated to what we were doing, and we enjoyed working with people, because we had seen such positive things happen. It was a real sad day in our lives when we were forced to stop. We had patients that were getting better every day, and they had to stop their treatments."

Dr. Mayer said, "It was a ruthless way of doing things."

"Yes," Joe continued, "it was very ruthless. I don't know why they chose to do it that way. But I do know that one of the individuals who complained knew a very influential individual in the FDA, and at his urging, this person at the FDA was able to do it the way he did.

"Normally, if someone was using a product that there was a question about it, the FDA would send in a team of two or three people. They'd come to you and say, 'What do you do? What is your reason for doing it? What is your authority for doing it? Do you have an ID with us? Do you have a study progress with us?' And if you answer no or you can't answer their questions, then they are going to stop you from doing it, and they may go ahead and prefer charges against you. That's the normal way of doing it. Well, that's not what they did with us.

"They turned it over to the criminal division, and they came in here with their guns drawn and put everybody against the wall. The criminal division deals with people who are making cocaine in their bathtubs or heroin or whatever, and this is the kind of treatment they would normally get, because they were very rough, they were very aggravating to the people.

"The investigator that headed this thing up was very belligerent to some of the people, including the one I told you about who was able to sit up and read his newspaper. They wanted to take him off the IV immediately. He said, 'You're not touching me,' and refused to let them touch him. And the guy said, 'This is going to be the last treatment you'll ever get.' And he replied, 'If that's true, then

I'm going to die.' And the guy turns back on him and said, 'That's not my problem,' and walked away. Very, very bad."

Albarin did not save my daughter, Sybil, but it did save many, one of whom lives today only twenty-two miles from my home. I recently talked with the man, a well-known gospel singer, and his wife. Oncologists gave him a death sentence, telling him he had only six months to live in 2001. He went to Joe originally after hearing of Sybil's case and talking with my son-in-law, Bill, about the clinic.

Dr. Mayer and Joe had a patient whose grapefruit-size tumor shrank under their care. She had been issued an ultimatum by her oncologist: she could choose either chemo or Albarin but not both. The oncologist told her she would not live longer than six months. She chose Albarin and was still alive a year and a half later. I do not know her condition today.

Deedy Fincher passed away on March 17, 2002, almost one year after Sybil passed away and five months after the clinic was shut down. She was a champion of Joe and Dr. Mayer until the day she died.

I recently inquired about the present condition of Pat's brother, Jim McEwen, and was told he was "doing fine."

In late July 2004, Teresa Crotts, Sybil's close friend, was diagnosed with lung cancer, but it was confined in one area. Her oncologist predicted over 90 percent chance of full recovery with chemotherapy treatments. When I talked to her shortly after her diagnosis, she was very optimistic. I spoke with her once again after she had her first chemotherapy. She was cheerful, fully expecting to recover completely. However, in less than two weeks, she was admitted to the hospital, gravely ill. The chemo was destroying her immune system.

She was slipping in and out of consciousness. Bud and Nikki were at her side when she started talking incoherently. Nikki asked her what she was saying. "I'm just talking to Sybil." Alarmed Nikki said, "Don't talk to Sybil now." Only a week later, Bill called to tell me that she had passed away.

It is ironic that Sybil was told she was beyond help with or without chemo, yet Teresa was given high hopes for life with the chemo treatment that killed her.

Dr. Candace Pert, a physician with Georgetown University's School of Medicine, writes, "Except for two forms of cancer, chemotherapy does not cure. It tortures and may shorten life—no one can tell from the available data."

Professor Georges Mathes, a French cancer specialist, said, "If I contracted cancer, I would never go to a standard cancer treatment center. Cancer victims who live far from such centers have a chance."

Allen Levin, MD, writes in his book, *The Healing of Cancer*: "Most cancer patients in this country die of chemotherapy. Chemotherapy does not eliminate breast, colon or lung cancers. This fact has been documented for over a decade, yet doctors still use chemotherapy for these tumors."

Alan C. Nixon, PhD, former president of American Chemical Society, "As a chemist trained to interpret data, it is incomprehensible to me that physicians can ignore the clear evidence that chemotherapy does much more harm than good."

I think that physicians of all specialties would do well to review what Hippocrates wrote in *Epidemics* (book I, sect. II):

> Declare the past,
> Diagnose the present,
> Foretell the future;
> Practice these acts.
> As to diseases, make a habit of two things—
> To Help
> Or at least Do No Harm.

The Albarin therapy helped Sybil's spirits and gave her quality of life at the end, and it did her no harm.

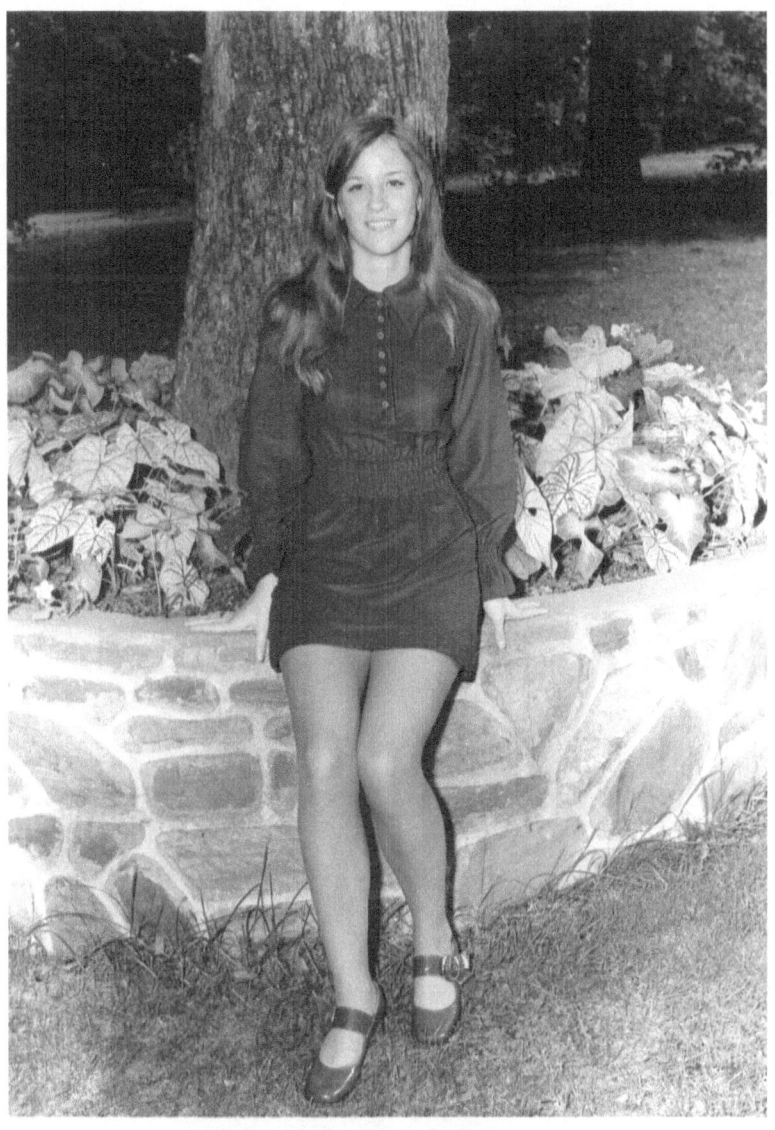

Sybil was the "Football Sponsor" on the
1971-72 homecoming court her senior year at
East Rutherfod High School; Forest City, North Carolina

www.ingramcontent.com/pod-product-compliance
Lightning Source LLC
Chambersburg PA
CBHW020917290526
45784CB00002BA/591